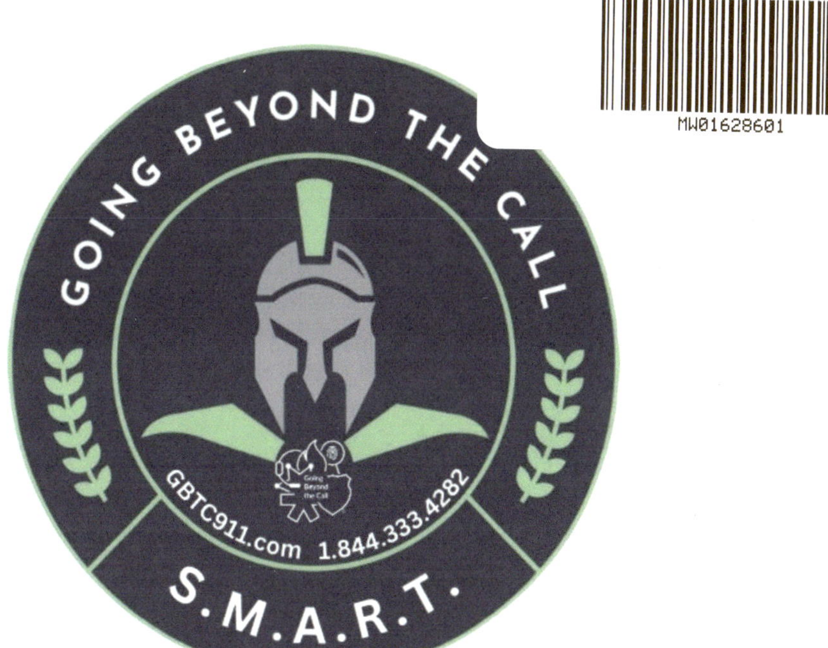

Survive the Mental Ambush Resiliency Tactics©

Workbook

Deirdre von Krauskopf
and
Sean Wyman

Follow us: https://www.linkedin.com/company/gbtc
https://www.facebook.com/gbtc911/

BOOK US FOR YOUR TEAMS: info@goingbeyondthecall.com

Going Beyond the Call Presents
Prepare for the Mental Ambush Workbook

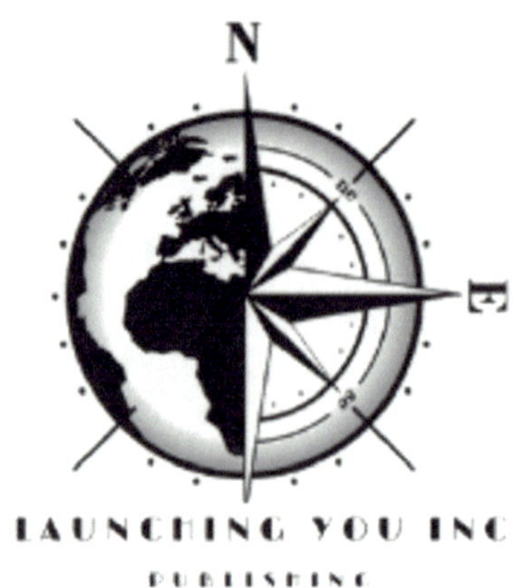

First Published in 2022 by Launching You Inc., Milton, Ontario, Canada
T: 1-844-333-7526

BULK PURCHASE: Please contact the publisher and author at:
info@goingbeyondthecall.com | **1-844-411-GBTC (4282)**

Logo Design: Lynn Wyman, Graphic Designer

Unnamed Graphics: Licensed through Pixaby.com

Editor: Valerie Cattau, CRPS

Researcher: Adam Karski, B.A.(Hons)

Book: **ISBN: 978-1-988995-25-0**
eBook: **ISBN: 978-1-988995-24-3**

SURVIVE THE MENTAL AMBUSH INTRODUCTION

Very few of you will manage a whole career without experiencing the direct, indirect, cumulative trauma and moral injury impacts of these high stress professions. Current recruit training identifies that it will happen, and you must deal with:

- Repetitive high stress incidents
- Personality, or behavior changes
- Higher than average addiction and suicide rates
- Poor health outcomes
- Relationships challenges
- Lower than average life expectancy

It is a common belief that these wellness impacts just come with '*the job*.' However, this is an outdated reality. Brain science and trauma-informed management has advanced to the point where organizational mindset needs to pivot to "next-practice" wellness. The benefits of our program will become clear as we prepare for and counterattack the looming mental ambush from all sides. The psychological, physiological, relationship, and organizational knowledge will change mindsets and performance at every level. In addition, organizations will experience fiscal improvements with our measurable trauma-informed training and practices.

This workbook is a companion to our book, ***"Going Beyond the Call ~ Mental Health Fitness for Public Safety Professionals."*** We have included a summary of each chapter in the following pages. Relevant chapters are referenced at the beginning of each major section for more in-depth learning. You can buy a copy of the book at *GBTCbook.com* or email *info@goingbeyondthecall.com* for discounted bulk orders. Connect with us for in-person or online workshops. Our two-day workshops include both book and workbook.

Our training is unique as we researched hundreds of journal papers, books, and interviewed leading experts to gain next generation practices. However, we won't bore you with academic lessons. Our workshops and material are presented in an easy-to-understand layman's perspective. Those choosing these professions are doers and leaders, not passive learners, so we present our material in a highly interactive and self-driven manner. Hundreds of testimonies rave about the Going Beyond the Call experience and we are thrilled to share self-directed adaptive resiliency tactics that will change your life. The pre-escalation or preventative aspect of our material will pave the way to a culture shift; away from the belief you must suck it up and live with the trauma impacts. We believe once we pivot the culture of individuals and organizations, we can all survive the mental ambush and serve our communities better while greatly enhancing our quality of life.

This workbook will guide a self-care journey and for some it will pave a path of awareness that professional support is required to heal. For Peer-to-peer programs and relationships, this workbook will enhance the peer training and offer conversational insights to help others in need. Organizationally, this work will benefit human resource management, personnel efficiency, fiscal responsibility, and risk mitigation. A resilient healthy public safety professional can better serve not only as the first line of defense, but also, as the first line of healing for self, peers, and the public served.

GOING BEYOND THE CALL ~ MENTAL HEALTH FITNESS BOOK SUMMARY

This summary won't provide the *'fill in the blank'* answers requested throughout the workbook however it will give you some quick insight on all the valuable information the book provides.

CHAPTER INTRODUCTIONS AS WRITTEN BY THE EDITOR:

In their introduction, co-authors Deirdre von Krauskopf and Sean Wyman cite the work as a manual for public safety professionals seeking solutions. Answers for the growing trend of unhealthy, unsafe coping behaviors, lawsuits, performance investigations, rising lost time budgets, decreasing mental health wellness, destroyed relationships, and ever rising tragedy of suicides among its members. This is accomplished through enabling individuals and organizations to mitigate the unavoidable trauma and moral injury impact of these professions, which will reduce self-harming and detrimental behaviors and the costs associated.

Additionally, utilizing the tri-faceted lens of psychological, physiological, and relational understanding, the authors can clearly lead the reader through steps of managing communications in potentially highly volatile and difficult interactions. They provide an understandable layman's grasp, for those who are new to the approach of basic neurosciences in human behavior, to lessen stress inducing situations and provide members with a powerful and groundbreaking 'pre-escalation' approach to communications. They strive to educate the reader about brain plasticity and how easy it is to develop and strengthen resiliency, "At any stage, rookie to retirement."

The journey begins with self and controlling the controllable. This includes a self-awareness and other awareness within peer groups and the public served for the signs of stress, mental health, and relational impacts. The exploration and instruction wrap up with the practices and an absorbable mastery of powerful communication methods. The expressed goal of this work is the mental wellness of the public safety community through the advancement of self- managed trauma informed adaptive resiliency. Building conscious competence on how to prepare for and survive the mental ambush in order to show up for their shift as the healthiest and happiest version of themselves. In short, this work addresses the need for a comprehensive learning that gets at the root causes of trauma and moral injury and provides actionable real-life solutions for successful outcomes. Further, it provides tangible tactics to avoid the common pitfalls and maladaptive choices that plague members that serve in high stress environments.

Chapter 1: It Begins with Understanding

This chapter begins by introducing the reader to the author's intention to educate on three key personal components to reducing the impact caused by high trauma professions. The authors also point out that cumulative stress build-up results in devastating and too often fatal consequences to public safety professionals, peers, communities, and homes. The beginning in the title refers to an acknowledgment that there is a crisis.
The understanding in the title refers to the need for public safety communities to understand the root causes of these challenges.

These professions are much higher in stress related health impacts, depression, PTSD, CPTSD, and suicide. Therefore, untreated stress disorders and mental fatigue lead to poor and failing physical health coupled with impaired decision making when both assets matter significantly on the job.

This chapter sheds light on the critical need for mental fitness training for recruits as well as annual core training. The public depends on these individuals to be prepared for repetitive traumatic engagement and the social/emotional challenges they must manage. While many agencies have improved peer-to-peer and critical incident supports the authors found no one adequately prepares their people for the mental ambush that coincides with their career.

Co-author Sean Wyman is quoted saying “preparation leads to preservation, procrastination leads to devastation,” a painfully obvious point when one looks to the career statistics that show only 3-5% of agencies have a suicide prevention program and most of those were implemented after the loss of a member.

With leaders like the authors sounding the battle cry for the mental health fitness and adaptive resilience of public safety professionals, leaders within these agencies are also finally recognizing the need for cultural change. Lastly, this chapter prepares the reader for the end goal of teaching public safety professionals how to manage themselves in a world where they are significantly impacting those around them.

Chapter 2: Stigma Busting

The chapter focuses on breaking down stigmas. Starting out the authors discuss why the current training standards cannot prepare for every scenario they will encounter. Next, they answer the gap with tactics a public safety professional needs to equip themselves with to create healthy coping mechanisms to prepare to face the repetitive cumulative stress challenges daily. By learning to manage their own stress and trauma injury impacts before attempting to address the stress and trauma of others they will lead with a pre-escalation mindset and avoid many escalated situations. The reader is warned of the risks involved of not facing the outcomes of untreated trauma and internal stress.

The authors speak on what is imperative to mitigating unexpected ambushes for these highly trauma impacted professions. This work seeks to encourage and even lead the way for organizations to create a trauma-informed culture where transparency regarding trauma and moral injury impacts is safe and encouraged.

The stigma that public safety professionals must swallow the pain and quietly deal with the internal storms caused by the situations and scenes they call upon is addressed. The reader will understand the value of being a trauma-informed professional.

Chapter 3: Why is Trauma and Mental Health Awareness So Critical

In this chapter, we explore approaches, practices, and instruction to reduce escalated situations and teach practitioners to effectively project their presence and communicate effectively in a crisis.

This can only be accomplished by developing a pre-escalation perspective. We also see why it is important to make mental health fitness a priority in our public safety organizations. Speaking clearly about their mission, the authors break down any lingering stigmas regarding brain sciences and medical outcomes that only serve to prove that the sooner someone deals with a traumatic event, the better it is for their personal health and the agency's bottom line.

Finally, the authors site the needed bridge between governmental agencies and budgets for equipping and training public safety professionals for self-awareness and community awareness which will only result in more successful engagement outcomes. When properly equipped and trained, public safety professionals will be more intentional in their interactions and be enabled to bounce forward with adaptive resiliency to traumatic events, experiences, and the effects on mind, body, and relationships.

Chapter 4: Understanding Trauma-informed Care

Most aptly defined, Trauma-informed Care and Mental Health Fitness is foundational training to ensure every public safety professional has the knowledge, tools and tactics to succeed personally and professionally within their communities." This chapter starts at the beginning - literally, childhood. Exploring A.C.E (Adverse Childhood Experiences) and their impact on the adults who live day-by-day in the shadows of their childhood experiences. This understanding creates greater understanding of the public served as well as opens one's mind to why we act and react to others.

The authors draw a clear line from untreated trauma in youth to an adult's responses to trauma around them, in the present. Shedding light on the outcomes of these communication encounters, also sheds light on the physical impact and ailments brought on by these trauma experiences, revealed later in life. Identifying these childhood traumatic experiences, unpacking them, and allowing more resilient management for oneself when one may have been pulled to this career due to childhood experiences helps with dealing with the trauma impacted public. It further wakes folks up to the unconscious and unknown health challenges associated with childhood trauma that gets further inflamed by the continued high stress, trauma and moral injury of these professions.

Chapter 5: Trauma-informed Care Outcomes

This chapter sheds light on the fact that trauma is a global reality, and that trauma is no respecter of age, gender, nationality, or time. The reader will learn how body language, choice of words, and emotionally triggered reactions, all play a role in the level of trauma to oneself and the reactivity of those around them. The reader will understand that to have command over a situation, they must first have command over themselves. The powerful communication tools, behavioral techniques, and personal examples from Sean Wyman's field experience in this chapter will aid public safety professionals in realizing better interactive outcomes, lessen threats and risk, and equip them to provide the best service in the communities they serve.

Chapter 6: The Body Toll

In this chapter, we learn trauma not only impacts mental health but physical health as well. The authors explain the value of trauma-informed adaptive resiliency and the benefits of mastering it. Through the author's eyes, the reader will see the first steps in becoming a trauma-informed professional. Then the authors take the reader through a higher perspective of trauma-informed care by evaluating the personal impacts to self, peers, the public, and families. The reader will be invited to learn the power of empathetic listening to foster and environment of safety, identification with the trauma of another, and provide a calm presence focused on the best possible outcome for all involved.

Chapter 7: Mental Fitness and Our Brain

This chapter provides insight into why a trauma-informed system will improvement the engagements with victims, offenders, and the public. The chapter also highlights the uniqueness of unveiling the underlying maladaptive human behaviors, which can be managed better from a conscious reality. The question, "Why is the rate of mental illness so high?" is addressed head-on. Relating back to the previous insight regarding childhood trauma, the reader will further see the correlation between childhood experiences, ongoing high stress, trauma and moral injury to the higher levels of maladaptive behaviors and illness in these professions.

The authors walk the reader through a scientific look at how the brain responds to trauma and stressed or triggering social/emotion human interaction. These insights reinforce living with unresolved, cumulative trauma results in intensified reactions which destabilize subsequent responses to stressful situations. Finally, the reader is equipped with pre-escalation techniques that prepare for the mental ambush and increase healthy brain responses. Tactics that both help individuals survive the trauma and moral injury associated with the job as well as help protect the public, they have committed their lives to serve.

Chapter 8: Stress to PTSD

This chapter begins by establishing facts that public safety professionals are exposed to a higher-than-average amount of stress, trauma, and emotionalized interactions. The authors reveal the signs and symptoms that self, family members, peers, and agency leadership should be keenly aware of when identifying and proactively addressing the often "vaulted" self-harming feelings and behaviors resulting from a career of horrific experiences. The reader will be able to identify trauma and moral injury and be equipped with an emotional X-ray machine for self-evaluation.

The authors explain that how one copes with trauma is critical in understanding the ways their own personal emotional escalations will be revealed in maladaptive behavior and coping mechanisms. The reader will be able to identify the early warning signs and symptoms of burnout and hypervigilance. The authors show the reader how to answer the question, "What does a traumatic or stress response feel like?" The reader will gain an understanding of how different responses impact performance on the job and at home.

Finally, the authors tackle the complexities of addiction in the section titled, "*An Introspection on Addiction*" Providing a new scientific way to understand the chemical elements of addiction versus the often-believed perception.

This will provide great insight as to how public safety professionals can successfully avoid harmful self-medicating and find healthier self-directed healing for their daily lives.

Chapter 9: Can We Do Something About the People

A key component to trauma-informed organization is the shifting of public safety professionals focus away from, "*What's wrong with you*?" to "*What happened to you*?" In order to more effectively understand how we got here; the authors take us back to the industrial revolution and show how the cultural shift to a transactional world started. Understanding how transactional versus transformational engagement and communications impact, both personally and in the line of duty, is critical in turning the Titanic of dealing with trauma in a proactive way.

10: Communications Gone Wild

In this chapter, the authors explore improving relationships by improving communication effectiveness. Stating that the cornerstone of effective communication is the projection of oneself as a calm, safe, and confident presence, intent on achieving the best interactive outcome, the authors highlight the role of humility as this mindset develops. Diving deeper into successful communications, the authors point out that another benefit of improving one's communication skills and emotional intelligence is the ability to engage with intentionality. The reader will see that people who cultivate and strengthen their emotional intelligence are better equipped to control their emotional responses, while influencing and managing others. Finally, they will see the role of listening in effective communications to create a common ground of understanding.

Chapter 11: Emotional Control and Contagion

In this chapter, the reader will discover the definition of "emotional or behavioral contagion." The reader will learn how to engage with highly charged groups in a way that accomplishes desired outcomes. The authors introduce the reader to "emotional control" and explain the benefits of mastering this skill with thorough practical evidence. Finally, the reader is shown the way to utilize the natural tools afforded each of us by our brain, to effectively manage themselves and those they are called to serve.

Chapter 12: Communicating with Humans: The Struggle is Real!

In this chapter, the authors identify why most humans communicate more successfully when they find common ground. The reader is then provided an effective, pre-escalation strategy for most of their calls. The authors demonstrate through accredited evidence that humans respond with the least escalation and unchecked emotion when this strategy is understood. The reader will also understand when it is safe and when it is not safe to apply these tactics. In providing the reader with an example of this dynamic, the authors highlight the mindset of bullies by showing the common influence of their past and how that drives their behaviors in the present.

Finally, the authors show the impact of ego in positive and negative outcomes, leading the reader to identify emotionalized ego indicators in themselves and those they serve both at home and on the job.

Chapter 13: Me Affects Thee

In this chapter, the reader will see the harnessing of ego in action and how it is best utilized for positive outcomes. The old Cherokee story is recast with its original meaning, which is quite different from what has been taught in modern times. The reader will understand the healthy balance between the light and dark side of ego and how they both must be balanced and healthy to sustain inner peace.

In picturesque fashion, the authors draw a close and impactful comparison between martial arts philosophies and the tactics taught in this book. The reader will understand the energy of emotions/words and how to redirect that energy to diffuse situations. The reader will also see the value of calmness in high tense situations and the power of body language techniques. The chapter wraps up with the understanding and application of internal and external focus in managing and influencing others.

Chapter 14: Complications in Communications

This chapter is the place where tools begin to be placed inside the toolbox for daily practice and use. The reader will learn tactics of "self-talk" and preparing oneself for calm engagement. All facets of communications are examined including body language, voice tone, pitch, and volume. The best and most calming use of these in emotionally charged situations is examined. The authors stress the importance of two key factors in communications for the benefit of those with whom public safety professionals engage. Finally, the reader learns why, while in a difficult or investigative conversation, there is great value in stimulating interest by creating a compelling "*What's in it for them*" message. Further, ensuring an environment of safety where both sides will be heard, understood, accepted, and respected benefits their conversational objective far greater than the typical authoritative approach, when safe to do so.

Chapter 15: Overwhelmed with Overwhelm

Humans are already overwhelmed when embroiled in a high intensity situation. When public safety professionals realize this in advance, the objectives can be set, interests stimulated, and safe environments ensured for conversation. In this chapter the authors address emotional management, encouraging the reader towards self-mastery. Public safety professionals are shown the value of extracting themselves from unhealthy emotionalized reactions that do not serve healthy objectives. Instead, becoming the one who brings the calm and safety to a situation by creating a rapport and establishing common ground. The authors lead the reader to see that a humble strength that aims to improve relationships and better every interaction is a power that is under control and comes from a place of authentic wellness.

Chapter 16: Emotional Intelligence: Me Factor

Skillfully and practically, the authors reveal the 4 quadrants to understand emotional intelligence. The reader will understand how Emotional Intelligence (EI) and Social Intelligence (SI) makes public safety professionals aware of others' emotional states and help them skillfully use their emotions for personal development and for influencing and leading others.

Public safety professionals are encouraged to develop their emotional quotient (EQ), equipping them to increase their ability to influence and inspire others while managing themselves more effectively. The authors also discuss keys to successful communication with intentionality. Finally, because public safety professionals have confessed that empathy is a challenge, the authors provide the reader with tactics to develop this crucial skill.

Chapter 17: Communication Power Tactics

This chapter teaches the reader to develop intuition skills. Public safety professionals will learn how to use intuition to improve situational awareness and environmental control as well as recognizing potential risk factors in those surroundings. The reader will also learn about three types of doors in communications and the strategies to gain access. Finally, the authors provide *power questions* to aid in facilitating deeper conversations.

Chapter 18: Emotional Intelligence Control

Here, the authors delve into a bit more brain science. Touching on the RAS (Reticular Activating System), the reader is led to understand the role of the brain in daily life, relationships, and responses to others. Through the rich content in this chapter, public safety professionals will be taught to control parameters and to prioritize filters in order to gain opportunities, meet people, and gain information that moves them towards mutually desired objectives. Finally, the authors address the extremely important roles of self-management, self-discipline, and self-esteem in emotional control, and how each one impacts the outcomes of engagement and effective successful communications.

Chapter 19: Personality and Ego States

This chapter deals with a brief overview of personality types and testing, often used in agencies to determine strengths and weaknesses. Then the more powerful psychological understanding of Dr. Eric Berne's *Ego States* is explored to share how personalities react and change when emotionalized. Stress and emotional reactions are explored under the lens of how they serve or hinder desired outcomes and recipient responses. Once the reader understands the Ego States, they can watch for patterns in others to analyze and adapt their communication approach. Being able to assess the Ego State one is faced with allows a pre-escalation mindset that is in control during challenging and emotionalized interactions. With brain armor in place, we can better manage and influence the conversation to the best possible outcome for all involved. The reader will also learn to avoid being triggered and how to redirect the conversation using the tactics shared in this chapter to move people away from their emotional responses.

Chapter 20: Take the Drama out of Trauma

In this final chapter, the authors lay the groundwork of how emotions impact our communication as they go deeper into the Ego States and our interactive success. This will allow the reader to start managing pattern exchanges that seem to trigger and loop into unhealthy relationships or repeated arguments with certain people or personalities. Readers learn the negative outcome of denying human interaction and attention. Strategic questions and messaging are also beneficial in reaching desired outcomes.

Finally, reviewing the use of transactional analysis in both favorable and unfavorable outcomes is a valuable tool in preparing the public safety professional for future engagements with intentional objectives and successful outcomes.

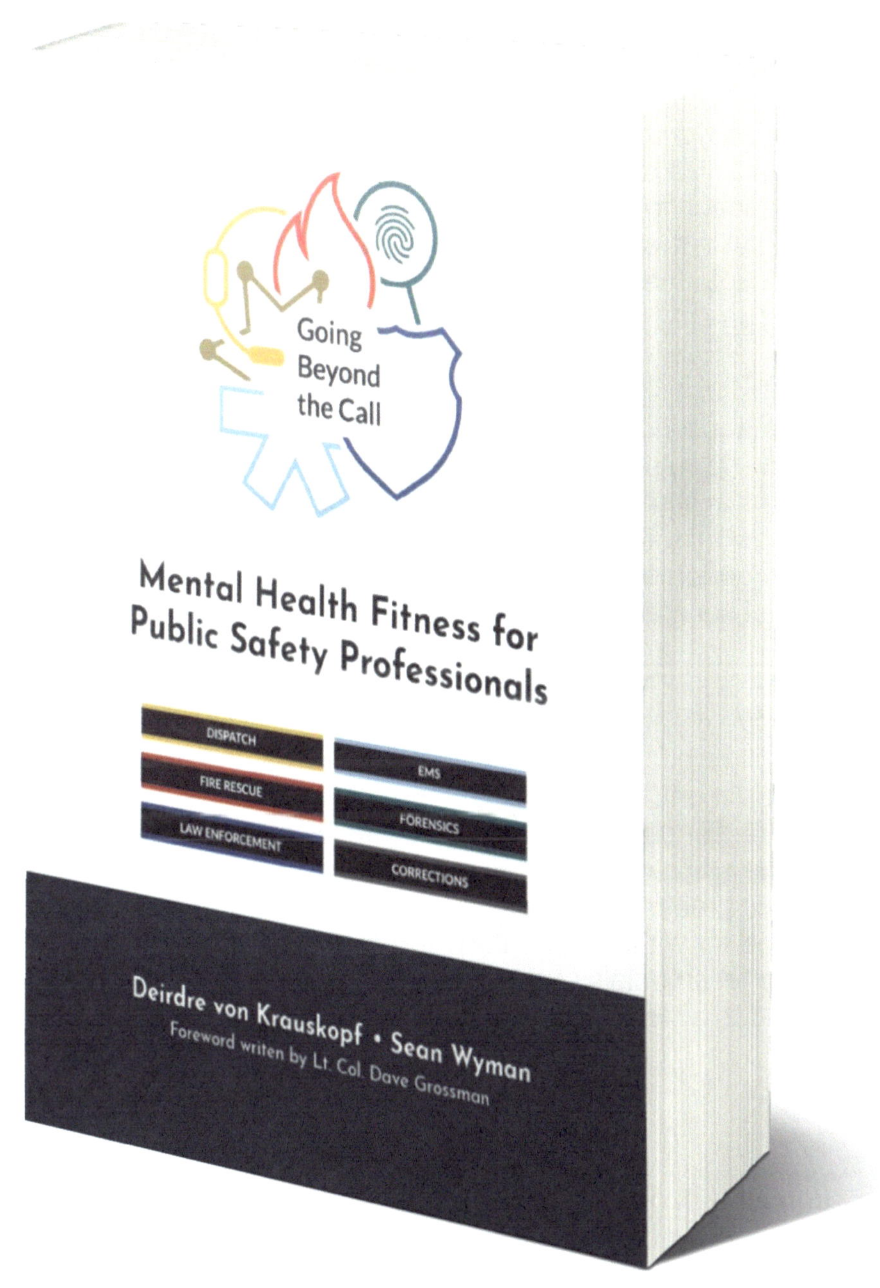

ABOUT THIS WORKBOOK

This workbook is a companion to our 2-day ***Going Beyond the Call ~ Mental Health Fitness for Public Safety Professionals*** workshop. The material in our workshop is based on our foundational work in the book of the same name, available at GBTCbook.com. Some content comes directly from the many customized seminars we have created since writing our book.

Please visit us at **GTBC911.com** and follow our Facebook and LinkedIn page **@GBTC911**.

We adapted this workbook to sell publicly to academies, colleges, and organizations. Given the highly interactive and demonstrative design of our workshops, there was a lot of blank space for attendees to write based on the exercises and presentations. Some of you may buy this along with the book with or without the online video series. We have added excerpts from both the book and workshop to help you align the teaching materials to the worksheets. You may read the chapters identified or watch the segments and journal as you go.

The original manuscript for the book was over 940 pages, so we have a lot of fantastic material to pull from, plus research we didn't include in the first draft. Our goal is to create a series of books aimed at serving many professions. I was initially surprised by how many corporations asked us to incorporate our trauma-informed segments into customer service and people engagement workshops given the overwhelming stress many folks have faced during the past couple of years. Check out our other corporate and public courses at DvKPartnerGroup.com and GoingBeyondTheCall.com.

To date we have created workshops, seminars, and speech content for many fields [educators, child welfare, students, health services, medical, military, manufacturing, banking, government, disaster relief, and other corporate professions], along with relationship weekends, public, and family inclusive events. The core content remains the same while the statistics, interactive exercises, and stories change. Our passion for serving the public safety realm first came from our personal experiences with trauma, and with those we cared for within the military and first responder ranks but it has grown due to overwhelming testimonials stating how transformational the content it, even from those who were voluntold to attend a workshop!

Please connect with our social media and send us an email with your comments, testimonials, and feedback for future editions. Have a question or wish to discuss a topic further? We would love to hear from you!

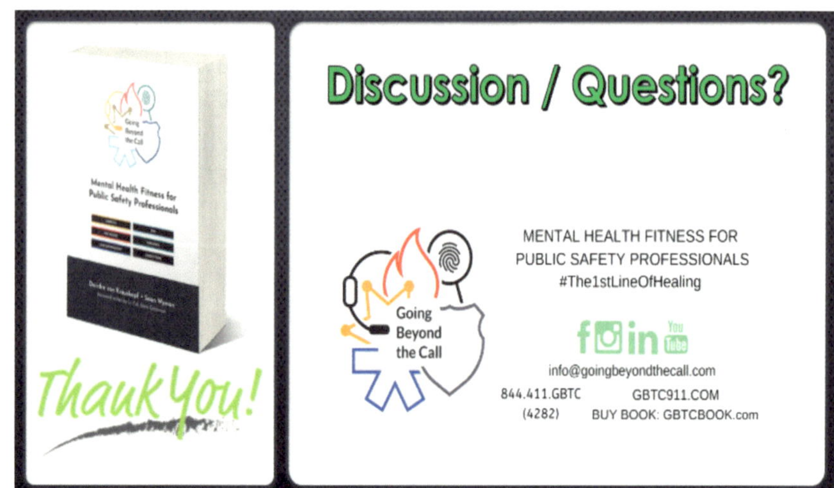

YOUR WELLNESS MATTERS TO US

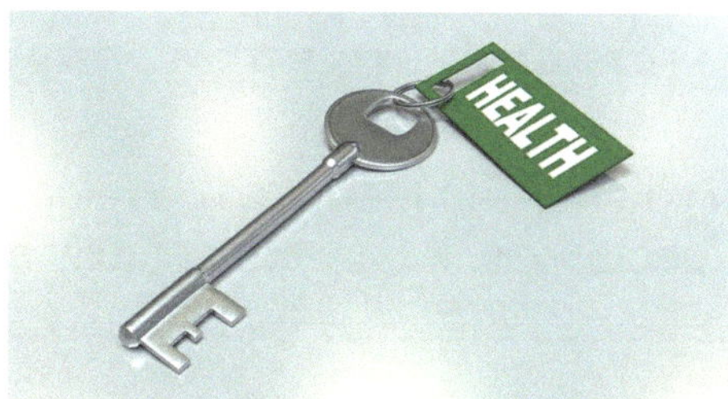

"I beg you take courage.
The brave soul can mend even disaster."
~Catherine the Great

We recognize the subject matter of this workshop, book, workbook, and/or video series may uncover some visual, sensory, and cellular feelings and emotions for those with trauma histories.

If you need to:

- Take a moment. If in our workshop, give us a nod and step out. If watching online or reading, stop, take a pause, and utilize a calming technique. A great one is two quick breaths through the nose followed by a longer sigh through the mouth.
- Be comfortable asking us to help identify a peer or professional to help you find the right support(s). We have collected a lot of local and national connections to share, including several psychologists who are familiar and supportive of our work.
- Practice tactical breathing – take a deep breath in; hold for count of 4; slowly breathe out for a count of 4; hold for a count of 4. Repeat.
- Chug water to help calm stress response. This tactic requires you to take a breath, holding it to drink, then breathe out.
- We are not clinical psychologists, that is what makes us unique. We present and share from a layman's perspective to provide foundational knowledge that will help you with self-care, or recognize you need support until you bridge to the point of self-care again.

Always seek professional help if you feel you cannot manage your thoughts or actions well on your own!

Do I have connections to an understanding friend or family member I trust, a peer, or health professional I can reach out to in a dark moment? If not, check the back of this workbook for options that work for you.

My 'GO-TO' human when emotionally stressed: ______________________________

My 'BACK-UPS: ___________________________ ________________________

"Once we accept our limits; we go beyond them."
~Albert Einstein

MENTAL FITNESS - CAREER - PERSONAL LIFE

What do you hope to learn and develop by the end of this program? Take a moment and set some expectations. If they are not fully met, then reach out to us and ask for further insights.

____

____

____

PSYCHOLOGICAL TRAUMA

(Read: GBTC book Introduction, Chapters 1-3)

What does trauma injury mean to you?

____

____

TYPES OF PSYCHOLOGICAL TRAUMA

1. ______________________
2. ______________________
3. ______________________
4. ______________________

"A lot of first responders feel that mental health help is almost like a trap.
They would rather just suck it up and deal with the consequences."
~Sean Wyman

STATUS QUO:

What percentage of training does your agency put towards core training versus the percentage of time towards managing the social/emotional aspects of dealing with people in their worst possible moments?

TRAIN FOR HIGH RISK/WORST CASE SCENARIO: ________ %

TRAIN FOR SOCIAL/EMOTIONAL INTERACTIONS: ________ %

Now in reality what percentage of time do you perform the high risk, urgent core training aspects of your job versus the social/emotional challenges of dealing with peers and people in distress?

____

____

____

What stigma is common in your workplace? Is it more top down, or lateral? How is mental health wellness perceived within your peer circles?

____

____

THE HIERARCHY OF SKILLS COMPETENCE (Source: Noel Burch)

UNCONSCIOUS INCOMPETENCE ***You are unaware of the skill and lack proficiency***	*The individual does not necessarily recognize the deficit. One may deny the usefulness of the skill. To move to the next stage, the individual must recognize their own incompetence and the value of the new skill.*
CONSCIOUS INCOMPETENCE ***You are aware, interested, but lack proficiency***	*The individual recognizes the deficit of skill or knowledge and values new insights on addressing the deficit.*
CONSCIOUS COMPETENCE ***You can use the skill, but it requires effort***	*The individual has learned the new information or skill; however, concentration and effort are required to demonstrate understanding.*
UNCONSCIOUS COMPETENCE ***Performing the skill becomes automatic***	*The individual has had enough practice that the skill becomes ingrained and can be performed automatically. The individual may advance to coaching or teaching others the skill.*

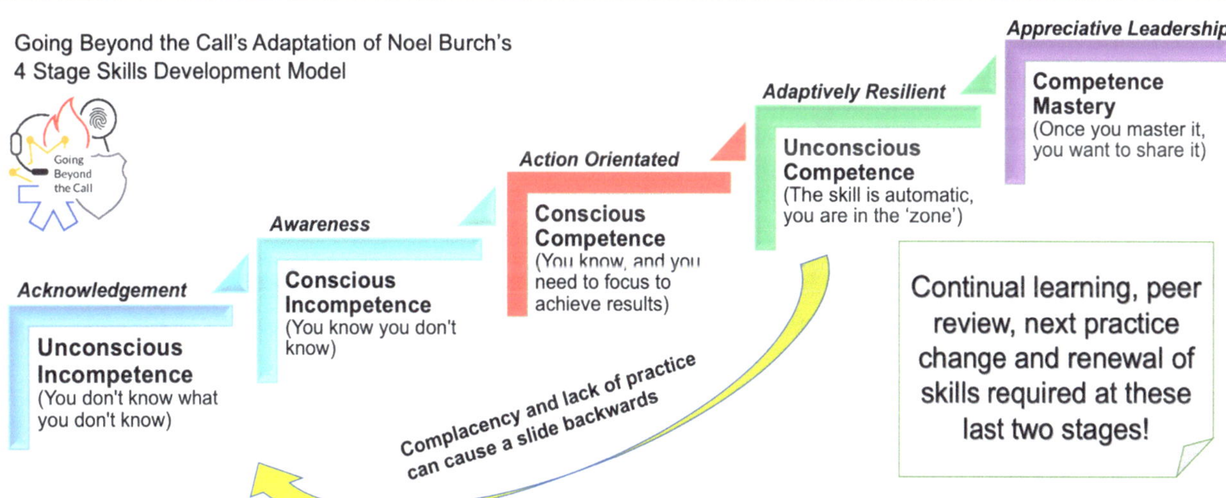

> ***"There is nothing noble about in being superior to your fellow man; true nobility is being superior to your former self."***
>
> ***~Ernest Hemingway***

We often fail to challenge our brains with new information, insights, and differing opinions. What are some of the areas I would like to build unconscious competence in?

____

____

____

____

A.C.E. - ADVERSE CHILDHOOD EXPERIENCES

(Read: Chapter 4 | Watch TEDx on Nadine Burke https://youtu.be/95ovlJ3dsNk)

The following are the *top 10* types of childhood trauma measured in the ACE Study by the Kaiser Institute and the Centers for Disease Control and Prevention (CDC) and Dr. Vincent Felitti. The most important thing to remember is that the ACE score is meant as a guideline for toxic stress under age 18. If you experience continued high stress inputs over months or years, then those are likely to increase your risk of poor health consequences.

There are, of course, many other types of childhood trauma beyond the top ten we see here. We have listed the next few that were studied on the following page. While reviewing this list consider the personal impact of all psychologically damaging events.

ADVERSE CHILDHOOD EXPERIENCE QUIZ ***BEFORE THE AGE OF 18***	**YES = 1**
Did a parent or other adult in the household often or very often swear at you, insult you, put you down or humiliate you? Or act in a way that made you afraid that you might be physically hurt?	
Did a parent or other adult in the household often or very often push, grab, slap or throw something at you? Or ever strike you so hard that you had marks or were injured?	
Did an adult or person at least five years older than you ever touch or fondle you or have you touch their body in a sexual way? Or attempt or have oral, anal, or vaginal intercourse with you?	
Did you often or very often feel that no one in your family loved you or thought you were important or special? Or your family didn't look out for each other, feel close to each other, or support each other?	
Did you often or very often feel that you didn't have enough to eat, had to wear dirty clothes and had no one to protect you? Or your parents were too drunk or high to take care of you or take you to the doctor if you needed it?	
Were your parents ever separated or divorced?	
Was your mother or stepmother often or very often pushed, grabbed, slapped, or had something thrown at her? Or sometimes, often, or very often kicked, bitten, hit with a fist, or hit with something hard? Or ever repeatedly hit over at least a few minutes or threatened with a gun or knife?	
Did you live with anyone who was a problem drinker, alcoholic, or who used prescription, or street drugs?	
Was a household member depressed, mentally ill or did a household member attempt, or complete suicide?	
Did a household member go to prison?	
Now add up your "Yes" answers: **This is your ACE Score:**	

BEYOND THE TOP TEN

Trauma-informed means recognizing the myriad ways trauma can be experienced and respecting the impact.

Beyond the top 10 ACE's the following are examples of trauma's that can result in major health challenges:

CHECK OFF THOSE THAT APPLY TO YOU:

Military Trauma	Juvenile System	Incarceration	Bullying	Traumatic birth
Parent Alienation (child(ren) or used to hurt co-parent or deny access)	School Violence or Group bullying (i.e., race, religion, sexual, orientation)	Victim/Witness to Community Violence	Serious Medical Procedures or Illness or Accident	High exposure to media, TV, video violence at young age
Natural and Manmade Disasters	Traumatic Grief or Separation	Generational, Environmental & Societal Trauma	Forced Displacement	War, Terrorism, or Political Violence
Job requires causing injury, or restraint of others in course of duty	Repeated exposure to acts of violence, or bodily distress on and in others	Repeated exposure to death and human savagery	Repeated exposure to inhumane acts or in violence against animals	Recurring stress of harm, injury, or death towards self by others/events

Untreated mental and physical challenges grow in proportion to experienced trauma

What did you find most startling, interesting, or thought provoking about ACEs?

____

____

____

____

____

____

What impact do you feel the pandemic will have on the younger generations?

____

____

____

____

____

____

ACE's, TRAUMA-INFORMED CARE, AND THE COMMUNITIES YOU SERVE AND PERHAPS, A LONG LOOK IN THE MIRROR!

Trauma-informed Care means: "An adaptation of principles and practices that promote a culture of safety, empowerment, and healing for those impacted by trauma" ~ Substance Abuse and Mental Health Services (SAMSA)

Based on an updated study of 25 States and 144,000 adults ACEs are linked to chronic health issues, mental health illness, and substance use. At least five of the top ten leading causes of death have been associated with adverse childhood experiences, according to a recent CDC Morbidity and Mortality Weekly Report.
(Merrick MT, Ford DC, Ports KA, et al. Vital Signs: Estimated Proportion of Adult Health Problems Attributable to Adverse Childhood Experiences and Implications for Prevention — 25 States, 2015–2017. MMWR Morb Mortal Wkly Rep 2019; 68:999-1005.)

WATCH: Everything you know about addiction is wrong with, Johann Hari.
https://youtu.be/PY9DclMGxMs

So, understanding ACE's and ongoing adult trauma can begin to sway our understanding of how people behave the way they do. It isn't always as easy as following the law, or just stopping a behavior that isn't serving us well. Addictions come in many forms outside of the illegal variations. Gambling, sex, food, alcohol, exercise, workaholic traits, electronic stimulation all fall prey to excessive use where we label them addictive. We aren't saying to stop enforcing or standing behind the law as it currently remains. However, we can deepen our empathy and comprehension of the addictive people we come across in the course of our duties. We can have a deeper sense of understanding for our peers that are caught up in self-destructive behaviors. We can look in the mirror with a little more honesty about our own challenges and be incentivized to make wellness changes.

"Addiction shouldn't be called addiction.
It should be called ritualized compulsive comfort-seeking*"
~Common Psychological Term

With this insight, do you now recognize any addictive type behaviors you fall back on when stressed or depressed that may have rooted from an adverse childhood experience? Is there a lack of connection in your life that often leads to unhealthy behaviors?

____

____

____

Can you think of someone in your life who suffers from a known addiction or perceived behavior that appears unhealthy and addictive?

____

____

____

With this new insight, do you have more empathy for the public you interact with when they are likely in the midst of a scared, emotional, or confused moment? What one new perspective stands out most to you when you think about how you have interacted with or judged someone showing signs of addiction?

____

____

____

Dr. Daniel Sumrok, director of the Center for Addiction Sciences at the University of Tennessee Health Science Center's College of Medicine states; "Since I've learned about ACEs, I talk about it every day." He also practices it every day, by integrating ACE's assessments for all patients in his clinics. He currently has about 200 patients who are addicted, most to opioids (heroin and prescription pain relievers, including oxycodone, hydrocodone, codeine, morphine, and fentanyl). "I've seen about 1,200 patients who are addicted," he says. "Of those, more than 1,100 have an ACE score of 3 or more."

What stands out to you as something you need to investigate further?

____

____

____

____

____

____

____

____

____

The WOW factor is real!

- *1 in 6 adults experienced 4 or more ACEs.*
- *61% have at least 1 ACE*
- *5 out of 10 of the leadings causes of death are associated to ACEs*
- *4 out of 5 Heroin users started out misusing prescription painkillers.*
- *ACEs of 4 or more lead to:*
  - *12.6% increase in coronary heart disease*
  - *14.6% increase in Stroke*
  - *24% increase in Asthma*
  - *27% increase in Chronic Obstructive Pulmonary Disease*
  - *5.9% increase in Cancer (excluding skin related)*
  - *15.7% increase in kidney disease*
  - *1.7% increase in lifelong Obesity*
  - *23.9% increase in heavy drinking*
  - *32.9% increase in smoking*
  - *44.1% increase in Depression*
  - *12% increase in suicide*

"What I'm saying is that early emotional loss is a universal template for all addictions. All addictions are about self-soothing. And when do people need to sooth themselves? When they are not being soothed." ~ Gabor Matè, author, In the Realm of Hungry Ghosts: Close Encounters with Addiction

Shoving emotions and psychological trauma in a "vault" doesn't serve you long term.

TYPES OF ADDICTIONS:

SUBSTANCE:	Alcohol, Pain Medications, Illegal Drugs, Nicotine, Caffeine
BEHAVIORAL OR PROCESS:	Gambling, Porn, Sex, Food, Shopping, High Risk, Exercise, Workaholic, Internet (Phone, Social-media, Gaming)

I MAY BE ADDICTED TO:

___

ADAPTED FROM THE AMERICAN ADDICTION CENTER (.ORG) QUIZ **Disclaimer:** *Only a medical or clinical professional may diagnose a substance use disorder. This assessment may serve as an indicator of a potential addiction but should not replace a diagnosis from a professional treatment provider.*	YES	NO
Are you worried about yourself or a loved one?		
Do you often use the substance in larger amounts or act on behavior over a longer period than you intended?		
Have you wanted to cut back on the substance or behavior for a while or had unsuccessful attempts to do so?		
Do you spend a great deal of time finding, using, making time for, sneaking, or recovering from _________?		
Do you have strong urges or powerful cravings to act on your substance or behavioral choice?		
Has your habit(s) resulted in your inability to meet your obligations at work, home, with friends, or socially?		
Have you had to cut back on, or abandoned social, professional, or recreational activities due to the habit?		
Have you repeatedly chosen to use or act on your habit when it was hazardous to do so, such as while driving a car or while working? Or, when discovery would damage your career, reputation, or livelihood?		
Have you kept using substance or acting on the behavior knowing that it has caused or worsened physical or mental health issues?		
Have you experienced social or relationship problems due to your substance use or behavioral habit and chosen to pursue it anyway?		
When you attempt to cut back on, or stop your habit use, have you experienced uncomfortable physical or mental wellness symptoms (withdrawal)? Or have you struggled to stop the pursuit of behavioral habit?		
Have you experienced diminished effects compared to the past and/or have you needed more of your substance or behavioral habit to feel the effects you're seeking (growing tolerance)?		
Generally, professionals look for the presence of 2 or more of these criteria being present in a 12-month period when evaluating for an addictive pattern. If you have 2 or more, please seek counsel.		

SAMHSA's National Helpline, **1-800-662-HELP (4357)** is a confidential, free, 24-hour-a-day, 365-day-a-year, information service.
https://www.samhsa.gov/find-help/national-helpline for substance and behavioral services.

SELF-CARE: NOTHING LASTS FOREVER

WATCH: YOUTUBE: Urge surfing: Meditation for cravings and impulse control https://youtu.be/imzq3p8Bxmc

Not quite there, but still a little worried about increasing cravings or habits? Urge surfing meditation for cravings and impulse control is used in some addictions treatment, in acceptance and commitment therapy (ACT), and in dialectical behavior therapy (DBT). Surfing helps control behaviors such as drug and alcohol use, emotional outbursts, aggression, and other unwanted impulses. The goal of this technique is to recognize and accept the feelings of an urge, rather than trying to suppress them. Relaxation and distraction are used to "surf" the urge until it fades away.

IT'S NOT JUST ABOUT ADDICTION…

Long-term impacts to physical health if prevention and mitigation actions are not taken.

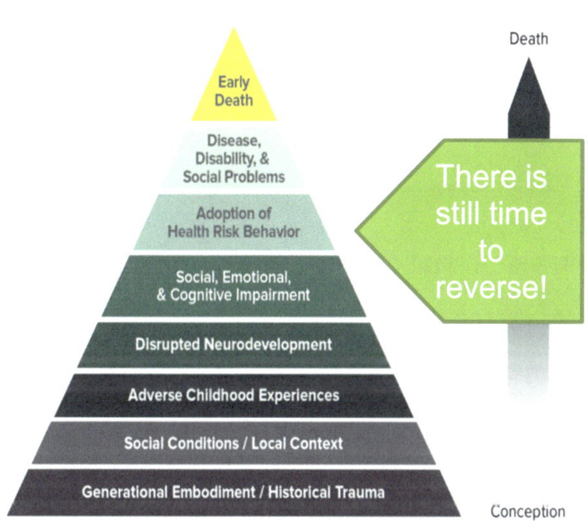

Mechanism by which Adverse Childhood Experiences Influence Health and Well-being Throughout the Lifespan

NERVOUS SYSTEM

Disruption to the developing brain, including changes to the hippocampus, prefrontal cortex, and amygdala, may lead to an increase in risk of cognitive impairment, attention deficits, learning disabilities, hyperactivity, self-regulation (behavior stoppers), memory, attention, and anxiety.

CARDIOVASCULAR SYSTEM

Toxic stress can increase a person's risk of developing high blood pressure, elevating levels of inflammation that can damage the arteries. These conditions can lead to heart disease, stroke, and other serious health issues later in life.

IMMUNE SYSTEM

Higher risk of infection and autoimmune disease may occur due to chronic inflammation and other factors, which cause changes in the body's natural immune defense responses.

ENDOCRINE SYSTEM

Toxic stress can impact growth and development. It can also lead to obesity and changes in the timing of puberty, as well as other issue

"Although the mechanisms may be different, addiction has many features in common with disorders such as diabetes, asthma, and hypertension. All these disorders are chronic, subject to relapse, and influenced by genetic, developmental, behavioral, social, and environmental factors." *McLellan, A. T., Lewis, D. C., O'Brien, C. P., & Kleber, H. D. (2000). Drug dependence, a chronic medical illness: Implications for treatment, insurance, and outcomes evaluation. JAMA, 284(13), 1689-1695.*

My take-aways for this section:

____

____

____

____

____

STIGMA (Refer to: Chapter 2)

Stoicism, Depersonalization and Derealization

Photo credit: © WorkSafeBC (Workers' Compensation Board of B.C.)

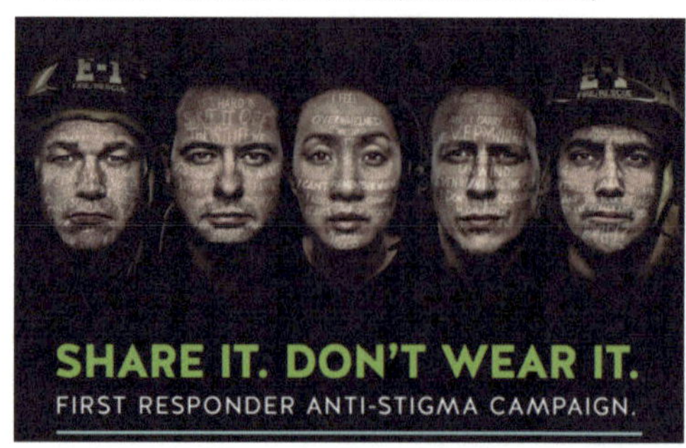

Stoicism, depersonalization and derealization are three common psychological defense mechanisms used by public safety professionals to deal with the wear and tear of the career.

Stoicism is a coping mechanism. A cultural expectation to hold it all inside, often manifesting as a dark sense of humor, which can be interpreted as cold and disrespectful by others.

____

____

Depersonalization is experiencing an event but feeling like it is happening to someone else.

____

____

Derealization is experiencing an event but feeling like it isn't real.

____

____

Many public safety professionals habitually use these defense mechanisms to cope with the occupational stress injuries from chronic trauma exposure not understanding these traits can become destructive both physically and psychologically. The habitual use of depersonalization and derealization can result in delayed onset of PTSD.

Those who bottle in toxic emotions are far more likely to cause themselves and others unintended harm. As we move forward consider the total health benefits to leading culture change by self-managing your wellness and supporting peers who are doing the same.

- Emotional Wellness is the self-awareness and acceptance of one's emotional reactions.
- Self- awareness in knowing yourself and your environment so that your emotional reactions appropriately match the circumstances that trigger them.
- Mitigate stressors by making positive choices and fostering positive relationships.
- Make conscious decisions to meditate, turn to peers, friends, and family for support.
- Developing effective problem-solving skills, keep a journal, or another effective stress management strategy.
- Creating a support network and avoiding those who may send you down a negative path.
- Understanding that a true buddy will build you up – not knock you down!

Peer to Peer support starts here!

TRAUMA-INFORMED LEADERSHIP

"If you don't want escalated emotional reactivity don't start it with your approach"

Ever wonder why that teen made such a bad decision? How about that young man from a disadvantaged neighborhood who seems to throw his life away in one bad day? When we layer in generational, historical, environmental, and societal trauma to other ACEs, we have a person deeply programmed and predisposed to bad decisions.

Changing your approach from "what's wrong with you?" to the trauma-informed mindset of "what happened to you?" allows professional empathy to be maintained. It gives meaning to why your approach should be strategic. Your choice of communication and body language have SUCH an impact on the response you get! When you provoke fear, pride, or confusion, you will almost always get an escalated emotive response. When safe to do so, ***Going Beyond the Call*** teaches a pre-escalation approach to avoid escalated encounters; some that may lead to career limiting actions or those that just add to another crappy day that follows you home.

Does this change your perspective on the fear-based responses your authority instigates?

____

____

ORGANIZATIONAL IMPACTS OF A MENTALLY UNFIT WORKFORCE

THE BOTTOM LINE

PEOPLE:
- Increase in complaints (internal/external)
- Decreased morale/cohesion/collaboration
- Challenges with recruitment/retention
- Trauma injury impacts to behavior/addictive coping

SERVICE
- Lower quality of service and proactive work
- Increased safety violations / protocol failures
- Erosion of focus, decision making, concentration
- Challenges with appropriate shift coverage

BUDGET
- Lost productivity (sick, leave, quit and stay)
- Lawsuits (public and hidden)
- Conduct unbecoming/disciplinary reviews
- Equipment repair due to lack of care/safety
- Recruitment/retention to department
- Administration/Leadership time investigating

AND

HAPPY HOUSE
HAPPY SPOUSE

In what ways does your organization support mental fitness?

____

____

____

TRAUMA-INFORMED ORGANIZATIONAL CULTURE

READ: CHAPTER 6

The 3 E's of Trauma

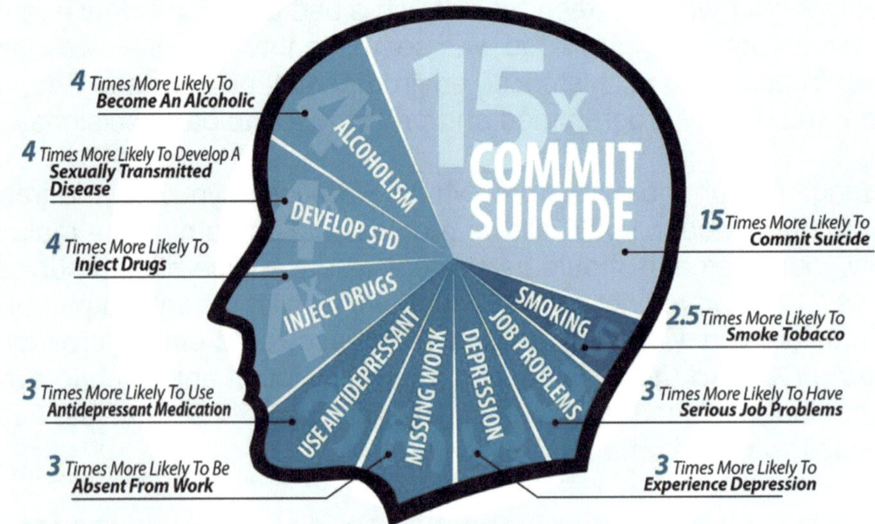

"An adaptation of principles and practices that promote a culture of safety, empowerment and healing for those impacted by trauma." ~ SAMHSA

EVENTS: Events and circumstances may include the actual or extreme threat of physical or psychological harm (i.e., natural disasters, violence, etc.). These events and circumstances may occur as a single occurrence or repeatedly over time.

____

____

EXPERIENCE: The individual's experience of events or circumstances helps to determine whether it is a traumatic event. What is traumatic to one individual may not be to another.

____

____

EFFECTS: Adverse physical, social, emotional and/or spiritual consequences. The long-lasting adverse effects of the event are a critical aspect of trauma and may occur immediately or may be delayed with short to long term duration where the connection to a trauma may not be recognized.

____

____

Examples of adverse effects include an individual's inability to:

To cope with the normal stresses of daily life	To trust and benefit from relationships
To manage cognitive processes such as memory, attention, and thinking	To regulate behavior; or to control the expression of emotions

TRAUMA-INFORMED CARE ORGANIZATIONS

Going Beyond the Call … Become the #TheFirstLineOfHealing

Trainees are not adequately prepared for the mental impact of what they will encounter on the jobs. Among the most troubling incidents are calls about child deaths, deaths of co-workers on the job and calls in which a person they help reminds them of someone they know. Emotional distress from traumatic experiences can last for years, especially if it goes untreated.
~Jeff Dill, founder, and CEO of the Firefighter Behavioral Health Alliance

How do you feel public safety fits into a Recovery-Oriented System of Care?

____

____

The Four R's from SAMSA along with Going Beyond the Call's additional 5th element:

A trauma-informed program, organization, or system that:

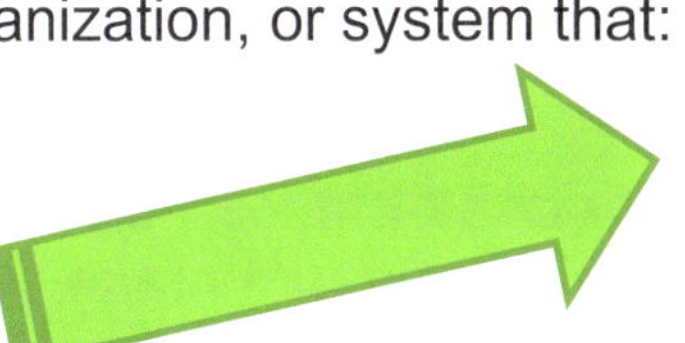

Realizes	Realizes widespread impact of trauma and understanding potential paths for recovery.
Recognizes	Recognizes signs and symptoms of trauma in clients, families, staff, and others involved with this system.
Responds	Responds by fully integrating knowledge about trauma into policies, procedures and practices.
Resists	Seeks to actively Resist re-traumatization.
Resilience	Resilience allows you to use tactics and techniques to build your defenses and healthy stress coping skills.

Going Beyond the Call has developed seven core principles to build an organizational recovery-oriented system of care within the public safety realm. Designed to help build agency statistics for budget approvers. Being able to prove a trauma-informed culture is beneficial for employee engagement, service enhancement, and budget improvement will go a long way to making mental fitness a core competency and training priority. Summarized here:

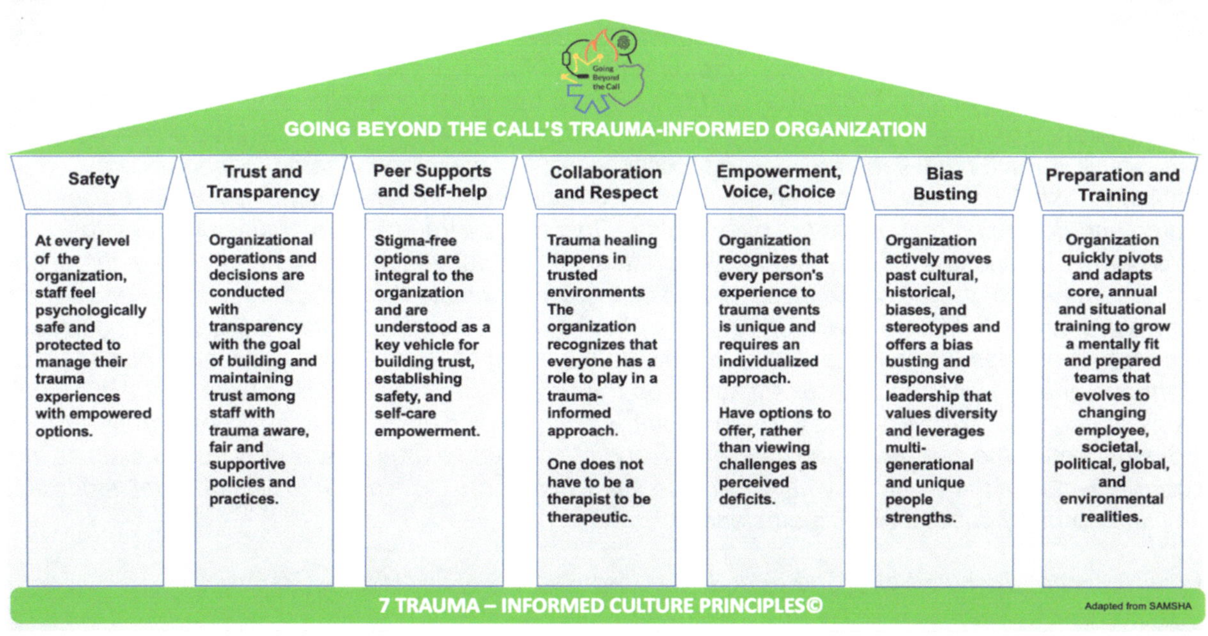

BRAIN MECHANICS 101
(Refer to Chapter's 2, 4, 6, 7, 11, 17)

Neocortex: Rational or Thinking Brain

Limbic Brain: Emotional or Feeling Brain

Reptilian Brain: Instinctual or Dinosaur Brain

Who's in charge?

Reptilian Brain's **4 F'S**

1. ____________________
2. ____________________
3. ____________________
4. ____________________

"It takes mental fitness training to balance emotions and logic. Most people when highly emotional lose their cognitive thinking ability. Conversely, becoming overly stoic and unfeeling you lose your caring and empathy. The goal is balance.

~ Deirdre von Krauskopf

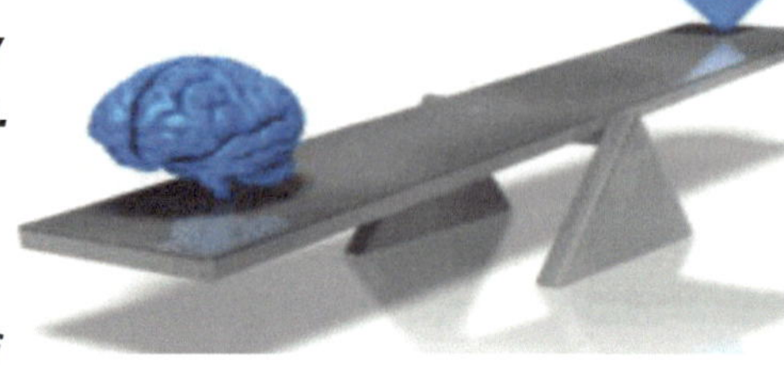

The more stress takes hold of our emotional or knee-jerk responses the less the cognitive neocortex is involved in our decisions. This is why smart people make really stupid choices they regret almost immediately after doing them. When has your Limbic (emotional) or Reptilian (instinctual) brains caused you to do something outside your desired behavior?

____

____

____

"In response to threat and injury, animals, including humans, execute biologically based, non-conscious action patterns that prepare them to meet the threat and defend themselves. The very structure of trauma, including activation, dissociation and freezing are based on the evolution of survival behaviors. When threatened or injured, all animals draw from a "library" of possible responses. We orient, dodge, stiffen, brace, retract, fight, flee, freeze, fawn, collapse, etc. All these coordinated responses are somatically based. They are things that the body does to protect and defend itself. It is when these orienting and defending responses are overwhelmed that we see trauma. The bodies of traumatized people portray "snapshots" of their unsuccessful attempts to defend themselves in the face of threat and injury. Trauma is a highly activated incomplete biological response to threat, frozen in time. For example, when we prepare to fight or to flee, muscles throughout our entire body are tensed in specific patterns of high energy readiness. When we are unable to complete the appropriate actions, we fail to discharge the tremendous energy generated by our survival preparations. This energy becomes fixed in specific patterns of neuromuscular readiness. The person then stays in a state of acute and then chronic arousal and dysfunction in the central nervous system. Traumatized people are not suffering from a disease in the normal sense of the word- they have become stuck in an aroused state. It is difficult if not impossible to function normally under these circumstances."

— Peter A. Levine, Author, Waking the Tiger, In an Unspoken Voice, and Healing Trauma

FIGHT - FLIGHT - FREEZE - FAWN (Chapter 7)

Watch: YouTube https://youtu.be/jEHwB1PG_-Q Fight and Flight response

The physiological impact of trauma, stress, and fear can get trapped in the body and we have a means to release it. As example, shaking or vibrating releases the chemical surges (like cortisol) and helps reset the body. In the public safety realm, there is a tendency to suppress and halt this natural release as we don't want anyone to see it and interpret it as a sign of fear. So hormonally juiced memories get 'stuck' in a spin cycle. Traumatic impact happens faster than we can cognitively process, and we need to counter that "hit" with any means necessary to reset our chemical and nervous system thereby prepared for the next mental ambush coming our way.

- Trauma occurs when the activated response to threat overwhelms the nervous system.
- The nervous system responds equally to trauma whether it is real or perceived.
- Trauma response is subjective and relative. Two people can have vastly different responses to the same trauma event.
- Traumatic events cause a disconnect between body and mind and the body. To heal you must create safety for your nervous system.

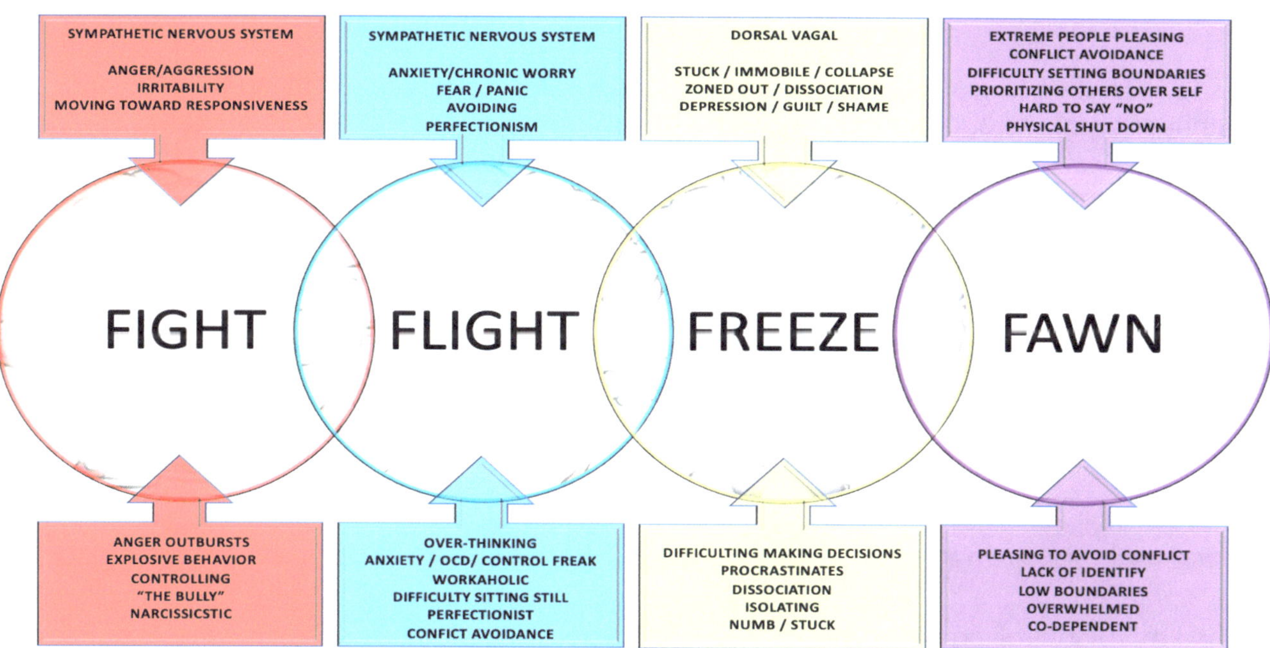

We can also have different reactions to different stressors or threats. Where do you see yourself in this chart compared when thinking of how you reacted on some of your worst days?

___

___

___

TRAUMA RESILIENCE (Refer to Chapter 11, 14, 15, 17-19)

EARLY ONSET RESET
HOW TO TAKE COMMAND & CONTROL OF OUR BRAIN

"The ingenuity of self-deception is inexhaustible," wrote essayist Hannah Moore in 1881. The act of rationalizing is so quick, the best you can do is to recognize when it occurs and choose to consider what else could be causing your reaction."

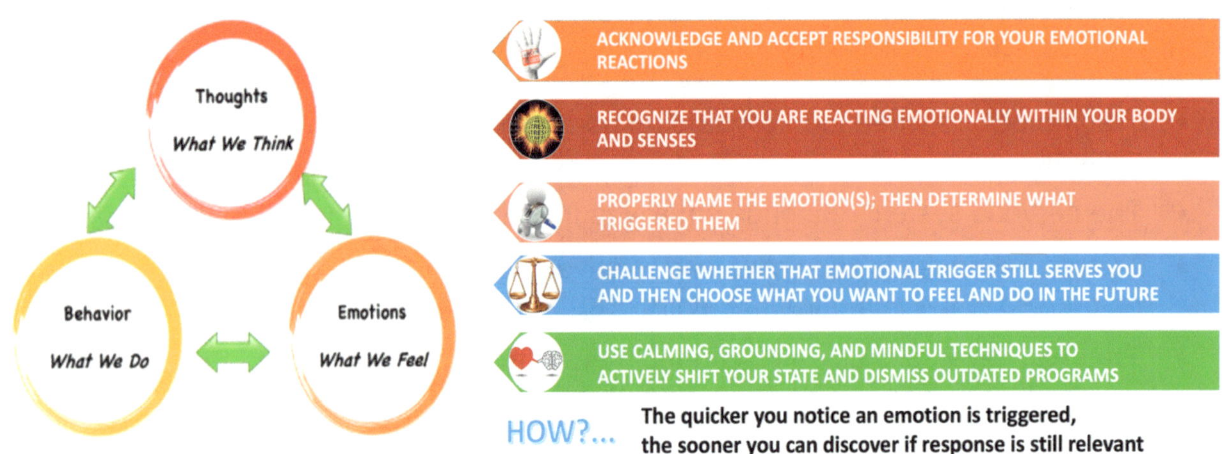

"IT IS WHAT IT IS" reminds me of a victim or defeatist mindset, just taking what comes without thought to our experience control or response options. I prefer to quote "IT IS WHAT YOU MAKE IT" as that is more active than passive and takes ownership and responsibility for our reactions and actions. By training our cognitive brain to take command of our reactivity we make better choices in our interactions with the public and our personal relationships.

How often do you release responsibility for aggressive actions, hurtful words, or self-sabotaging behaviors due to "the job" or "the stress build-up?"

____

____

CREATE CONTROLLED CALM (Refer to Chapter 19)

The key to controlling our reactions lies in conscious mindfulness. Being aware of our triggers and physiological changes allows us to counter with calming techniques when the moment arises. When we do not consciously take control of our autonomic nervous system, our subconscious mind will take care of everything for us, often using outdated and unhelpful memories and feelings to drive our actions.

Self-development helps us understand and manage our reactivity and provides control over the conscious and subconscious inputs we use to make decisions. This allows further control over our biological response. Here are a few examples with links to explore and build your mindful experience options. No one way works for everyone so investigate and find what works best for you.

BOX BREATHING e.g.: https://youtu.be/FJJazKtH_9I	HEALING CHI e.g: https://youtu.be/rpHy6hzNDI4	TREMOR RELEASE e.g.: https://youtu.be/xmn1BucNrzA
GROUNDING TO NATURE MUSIC e.g.: https://youtu.be/prfZFyp4XZk	ANXIETY BUSTER – 5.4.3.2.1. e.g.: https://youtu.be/cxflwM6YfYk	SELF REFLEXOLOGY DESTRESS e.g.: https://youtu.be/3yG72oz3eHc https://youtu.be/2Mu5RvPoOuo
MINDFUL EATING e.g.: https://youtu.be/eY54f3dyhcl	MEDITATION e.g.: https://youtu.be/Bw46jzi95yk	SNORE CANCELING SLEEP NOISE e.g.: https://youtu.be/oKuLSz0adiM
TAI CHI FOR FIRST RESPONDERS e.g.: https://youtu.be/0FvYlWXbuZI	PHYSIOLOGICAL SIGH e.g.: https://youtu.be/AjzdvO14OKU	NERVOUS SYSTEM RESET e.g.: https://youtu.be/rpHy6hzNDI4
YOGA FOR FIRST RESPONDERS e.g.: https://youtu.be/DYges5UqleM https://youtu.be/gQZhJIYTBR8 https://youtu.be/hBWo0h4wmis	MEDITATION FOR HATERS *Explicit Language e.g.: https://youtu.be/92i5m3tV5XY	PROGRESSIVE MUSCLE RELAXING e.g.: https://youtu.be/TNdEb8VeBF4

Journal as you watch and try these different options and share your thoughts on the benefits you feel. Which do you like, and which are not for you, or, not for you right now?

Your present circumstances don't determine your future,
They only identify today's starting point.

~ Deirdre von Krauskopf

MIND FULL OR MINDFUL?

(Refer to Chapter 6; Complete quiz on next page for area that may need a little attention)
Watch YouTube: Why Mindfulness Is a Superpower: An Animation - youtu.be/w6T02g5hnT4

Mindfulness is a form of self-regulating and taking control over our physiological self to be in the moment, situationally aware and cognitively purposeful.

WHAT RELAXES ME MOST?

____

____

____

WHAT AM I WILLING TO TRY?

____

____

____

Example exercise to use with peers when an event overwhelms the senses:

MINDFULNESS 5-4-3-2-1

5 THINGS YOU CAN SEE
4 THINGS YOU CAN TOUCH
3 THINGS YOU CAN HEAR
2 THINGS YOU CAN SMELL
1 THING YOU CAN TASTE

Socks of Doom Watch: youtu.be/3oKuvEgf7IA

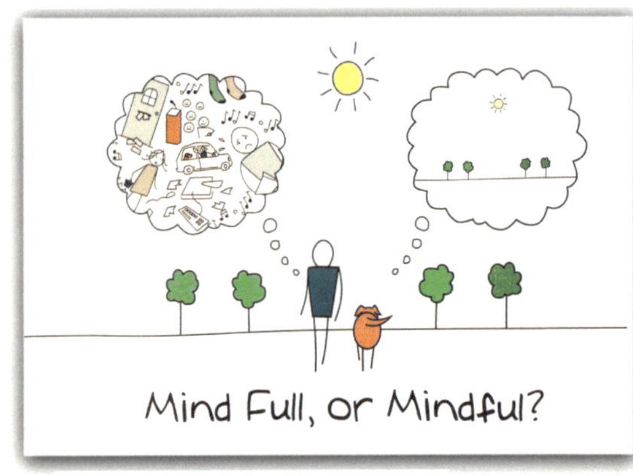

Art: Henck van Bilsen

Awareness to the known and acceptable stressors is one thing. Being brave enough to build prevention and mitigation tactics into your daily life means you no longer live under a cloud of self-deception. What is your support and stress relief system like? Are there areas you may wish to focus on to build them up?

____

____

____

____

____

"Challenge your mental fitness by learning to stay present in the moment. Not the past, filled with trauma memories, not worried about the maybes of the future. Mindfully present and open to the moment you are in … right now!"
~ Deirdre von Krauskopf

EMOTIONAL WELLNESS (Refer to Chapter 6)

What are my stabilizing roots – how much effort do I put into keeping them strong?

Mindful wellness starts with knowing where you are at. There is no right number to land on. This assessment allows you to take note of where your strengths lie and what areas you may choose to build upon or develop new root strengths to improve your internal wellness system.

The Big 7 Self-Assessment

On a scale of 1 (low) – 10 (high), rate yourself according to how **true** the following statements are when you apply each statement's significance to your life currently.

Circle the number that represents where you best fit on the scale

Family

I have a strong support network of related individuals whom I can lean on and go to for anything. We share experiences, learn from each other and share an unbreakable bond.

1 . 2 . 3 . 4 . 5 . 6 . 7 . 8 . 9 . 10

Career

I experience the utmost satisfaction from the work I do and the results that I produce and achieve daily.

1 . 2 . 3 . 4 . 5 . 6 . 7 . 8 . 9 . 10

Social Life

I have friends in my life that I can freely share my innermost thoughts and feelings with. Around them, I can be totally "Me". I can be "real".

1 . 2 . 3 . 4 . 5 . 6 . 7 . 8 . 9 . 10

Health & Fitness

I experience a high level of vitality and physical well-being. I practice good health habits, eat nutritious foods, get enough rest and relaxation, and exercise regularly.

1 . 2 . 3 . 4 . 5 . 6 . 7 . 8 . 9 . 10

Finances

I have the ability to create the wealth I need to fulfill my mission and greatest destiny. I earn the amount of money I need so that I'm not always worried about "money". I know I deserve to experience prosperity in my life…and I do!

1 . 2 . 3 . 4 . 5 . 6 . 7 . 8 . 9 . 10

Spiritual Journey

I am at peace with my current state of progress on my spiritual journey and I'm excited to experience continued clarity, growth and development as this journey continues to unfold.

1 . 2 . 3 . 4 . 5 . 6 . 7 . 8 . 9 . 10

Legacy

I feel fulfilled and humbled as I look at the legacy my life will be leaving behind. I'm always looking for new ways to leave this planet in better shape then I found it and I continually strive for opportunities to contribute and invest in the planet and in people.

1 . 2 . 3 . 4 . 5 . 6 . 7 . 8 . 9 . 10

Beyond the Big 7 Options to consider	
	Family
	Friends
	Peers
	Career
	Health
	Finances
	Spiritual
	Community
	Friends
	Love Partner
	Fitness
	Legacy
	Hobbies
	Social life
	Support Grroups
	Emotional Intelligence
	Learning
	Pets
	Love Partner
	Fitness
	Your choice:
	Your choice:

A big strong Oak tree can be felled in a night when the storms are raging, yet a Willow tree or Bamboo can bend all the way to the ground and bounce back after the storm passes. The Big 7 Assessment gives you the common options people turn to in times of stormy stress. It is by no means the only ones to choose from. Toxic relationships may mean substituting other options or developing new healthy and positive choices. There may be times different solutions are needed for wellness.

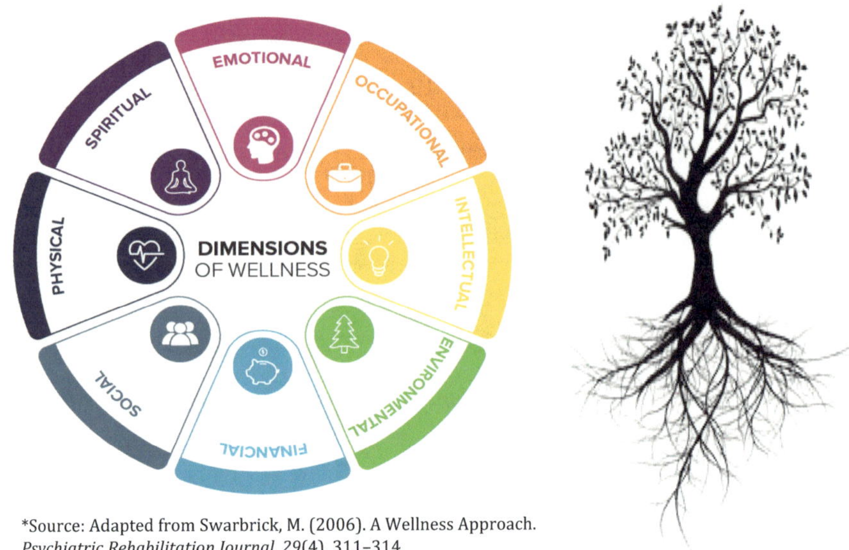

*Source: Adapted from Swarbrick, M. (2006). A Wellness Approach. *Psychiatric Rehabilitation Journal, 29*(4), 311–314.

The ability to adapt when emotional stress takes a negative turn and effectively cope with stress may not always be a quick fix. It starts with developing and satisfying your hierarchy of needs. You choose what is most important to you and build your coping roots, so they are strong and wide and well suited to handle the biggest of storms.

Based on my current insight on where I sit on the Big 7 (and beyond) wellness review what areas will I put focus on and develop?

GOAL	1ST STEP	BY WHEN?

Emotion: The word we use to describe feelings is the sensory responses to chemicals released in the bloodstream. With root system goals we take ownership of our reactivity because we have a plan to counter the sensory inputs.

MEETING PEOPLE WHERE THEY ARE AT

(Refer to: GBTC Chapter 18,19)

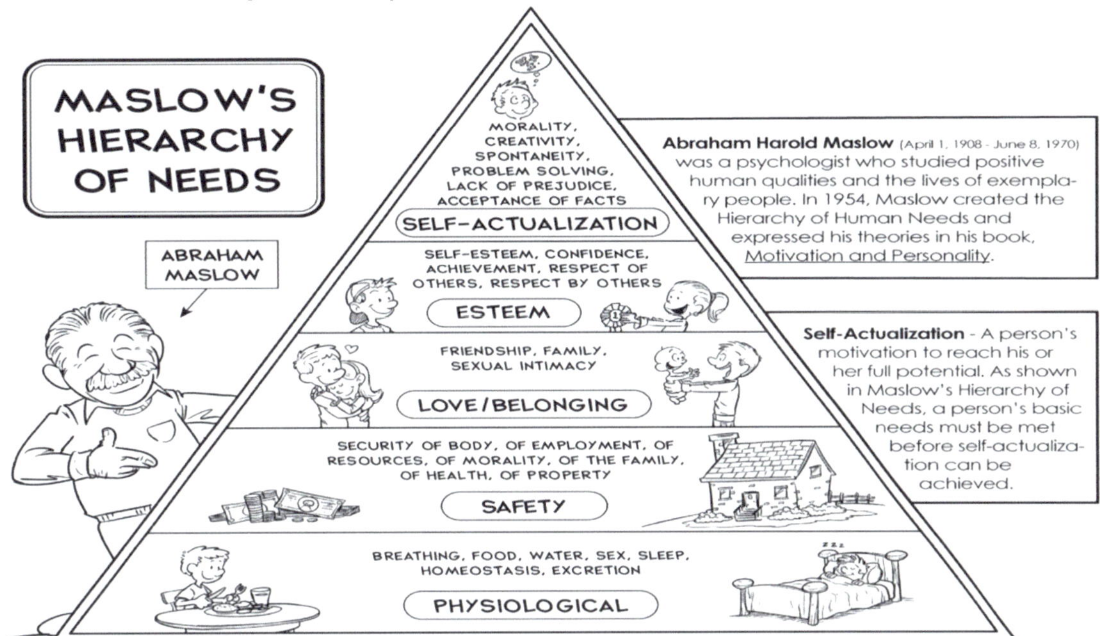

We slip up and down the scale of inner comfort, peace, joy, and security based on life events.

The environmental, social, and economical stress of the past few years has left few unscathed. Our youth's anxiety and depression are through the roof, and all people seem more divided than ever. Pandemics, rioting, war, mass shootings, family and financial stressors have taken a toll on our hierarchy of needs. Even the rebound aspect from social isolation have impacted how we act and react in the world. Is it fair to say all are impacted in some way?

How have the events of the past few years impacted you? Your family? Your friends? Your peers?

____

____

____

____

____

Understanding trauma-informed care means knowing that those most impacted will have significant stress build-up and more prone to acting out defensively, aggressively, and out of normal character.

Your pre-escalation approach in body language, communication style, choice of words can be one of safe strength, calm confidence, and mindful interaction. You cannot change another's actions, but you can change your response to others with your approach and your messaging!

LIVING IN A HIGH STRESS WORLD
(Refer to: GBTC Chapter 8)

RECOGNIZING STRESS TRIGGERS ~ SELF AND PEERS

Healthy Brain — Results of Chronic Stress

Front / Temporal lobes / Back

WHAT ARE MY TRIGGERS?

____
____
____
____
____
____

Anything that sets you off emotionally and activates memories of your trauma. Unconsciously, we are reliving feelings and behaviors from that time.

____
____

GOOD STRESS ... BAD STRESS .... AND HOLY CRAP STRESS!

IN THE LAST MONTH - HOW OFTEN HAVE YOU FELT? If majority fall to often and very often it is time to reach out for help! Source: psycom.net/stress to PTSD test	Never	Rarely	Often	Very Often
Repeated, disturbing memories, thoughts, or images of a stressful experience from the past?				
Feeling very upset when something reminded you of a stressful experience from the past?				
Avoid activities or situations because they remind you of a stressful experience from the past?				
Feeling distant or cut off from other people?				
Feeling irritable or having angry outbursts?				
Having difficulty concentrating?				

AWARENESS - PREVENTION AND MITIGATION
(Refer to Chapter 8)

We need stress! Good stress, or eustress, motivates us, gives us thrills, pushes our drive to accomplish things and helps us feel good in life. Bad stress, or distress, is what we want to watch out for. It can lead to so many mental and physical issues if we don't manage it well.

https://developingchild.harvard.edu/science/key-concepts/toxic-stress/

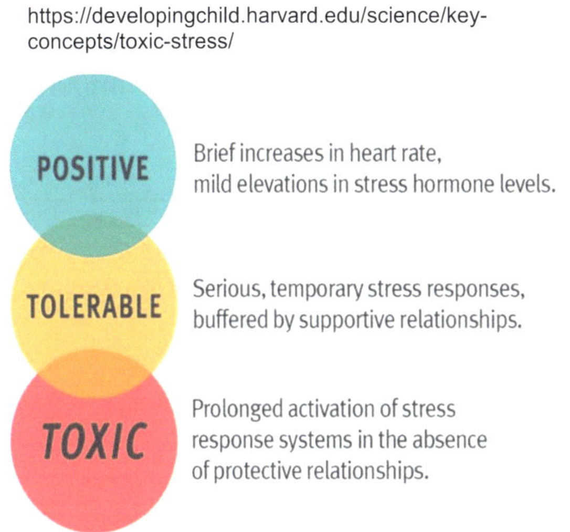

PNGkey: Yerkes-Dodson Model

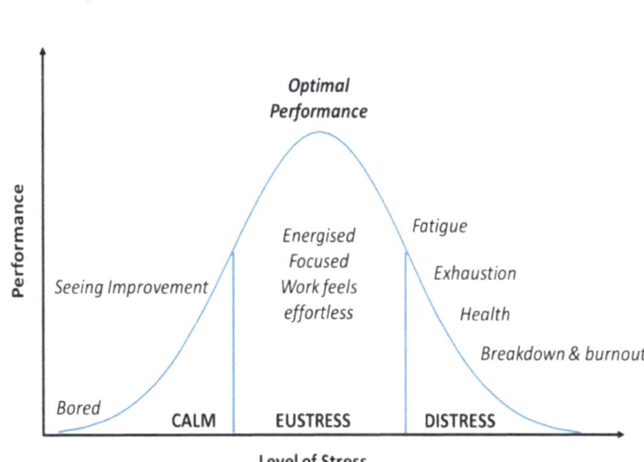

Where do you feel your stress sits on this scale most days? What are the main influencers to your negative stress? What are some of your positive stressors?

____

____

We will share ***Going Beyond the Call's*** adaptation of the Window of Tolerance. It was originally developed by Dr. Dan Siegel to describe the optimum zone of "arousal" for a person to function well in everyday life. It is a tool used in therapy to help people discover and grow emotional space; where they feel safe, comfortable, ready to receive, process, and integrate information in response to daily demands.

Since we know public safety professionals do NOT operate in the normal zone on a regular basis, we aim to grow your individual window of tolerance in this program using a new term we created called "adaptive resiliency©" You all come to this job with higher-than-average resiliency, notably called the "Bounce Back Factor" in most studies and literature on resilience the goal is using positive psychology to return to your previous state. This issue is in THESE professions, especially over time there is no bouncing "back" to who you once were. This is extremely important knowledge for personal relationships. Our loved ones also need to be adaptive resiliency to evolve the relationship to the new forms of you that will transpire.

Some will be able to create a larger tolerance zone on their own hence many happy, retired professionals with great stories to tell and healthy, lasting relationships. However, the statistics on depression, addiction, failed relationships, early death, and suicide also inform us many need more help in this area of emotional intelligence.

To manage the psychological and physiological stress of your experiences we must understand what happens during duress and trauma events and how to quickly respond to anxiety, exhaustion, trauma exposure, and feeling out of control emotionally. When we do not have this skill, our window of tolerance narrows.

There are two types of response (often not a choice of response), our body takes over and forces emotional reactivity upon us. It may show as hyperarousal, where you are anxious, angry, overwhelmed, and feeling out of control. It may show as hypo-arousal, where you are zoned out, numb, non-reactive, frozen, or the body just shuts-down. The narrower your window of tolerance grows, the less it takes to throw you off balance. Hence the cumulative danger of trauma in these fields. We build adaptive resilience when we can:

- manage the stress response and actively reset our physiology with grounding exercises
- do an introspective deep dive on how and why those reactive emotions are so stimulating
- have tactics in place to mitigate emotional response
- grow our emotional intelligence and communication skills to manage life's challenges

When we don't life gets messy, sort of like this chart, which visually shows when your window of tolerance is left untreated and unmanaged it can move beyond self-care and into trauma crisis.

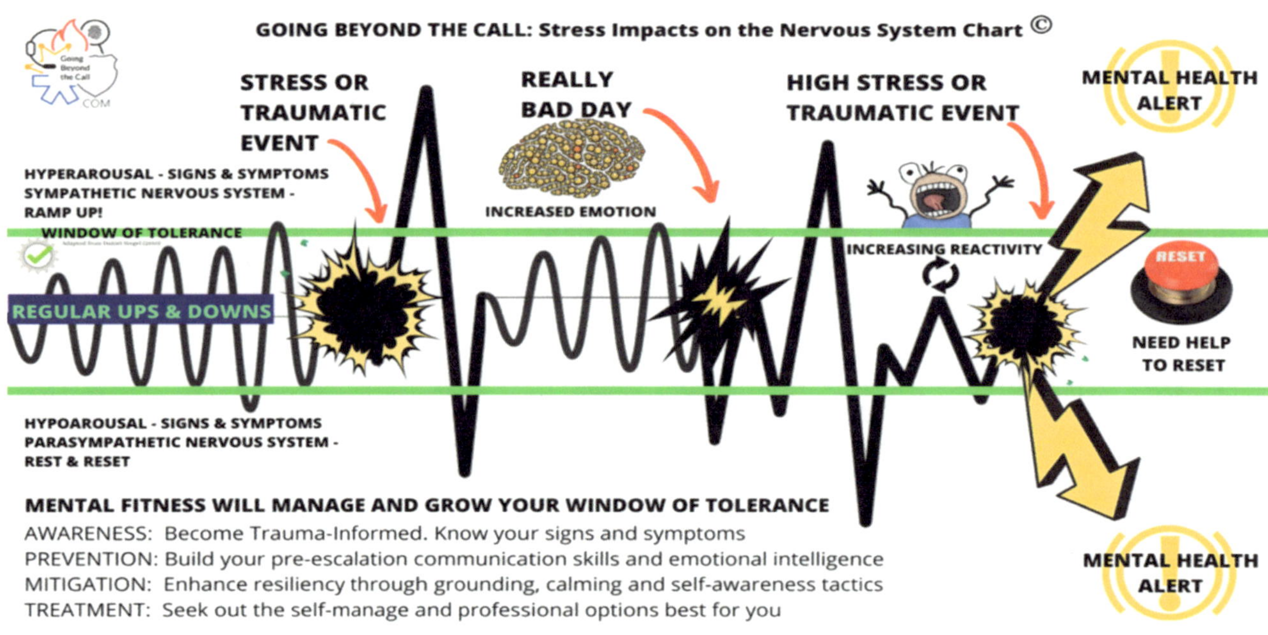

What did I learn in this section on stress that made me rethink how I view the emotional triggers I face on and off the job?

____

____

____

TRAUMA RESPONSE: A NORMAL REACTION TO AN ABNORMAL SITUATION

(Refer to: GBTC Chapters 7 and 8)

People may find that their relationships with others starts to change due to direct or repeated exposure to trauma. Sufferers may find they start to have difficulty in trusting others. One may become suspicious of authority figures and community leaders. Minor annoyances flare up into larger issues and often one just wants to be left alone.

Research into neuroscience proves there is a biological impact affecting the body during trauma. You now know the nervous system can be overwhelmed into fight or flight when a threat does not dictate it is necessary with a narrowed window of tolerance. Our nervous system and brain's response can lose its ability to differentiate between major, minor, and negligible arousal events. Even the most resilient can be impacted to the point they ramp-up or shut-down quickly and more often.

Our stress response system is powerful and critical in threat situations. However, it wasn't intended to be activated regularly and repeatedly. This heightened cycling has serious adverse impacts on our mental fitness, long-term physical health, as well as with all our interactions and relationships. ALL trauma-based injuries i.e., burnout, depression, hypervigilance, PTSD, C-PTSD, have some combination of hypo or hyper behavior, physical, cognitive, and emotional reactions, as shown in this chart below. Whether you are a leader or peer, this snapshot of signs and symptoms can be used to identify behavioral changes in others, and when we are honest enough, within ourselves. Understanding the stress tolerance model allows us to see where we default to.

YOUR TRAUMA EXPERIENCE CHECKLIST WHAT HAPPENS TO YOU AFTER A TRAUMA EVENT? HOW ABOUT MONTHS/YEARS LATER?							
EMOTIONAL		COGNITIVE		BEHAVIORAL		PHYSYCAL	
EMOTIONAL SHOCK		POOR PROBLEM SOLVING		STARTLE REFLEX INTENSIFIED		RAPID HEART RATE	
APPREHENSION		INCREASED OR DECREASED SITUATIONAL AWARENESS		CHANGE OF COMMUNICATION STYLE		DIFFICULTY BREATHING	
LOSS OF CONTROL		HYPER-VIGILENCE		CHANGE IN ACTIVITY LEVEL +/-		ELEVATED BLOOD PRESSURE	
OVERWHELM		MEMORY PROBLEMS		ANTISOCIAL ACTS		DIZZINESS / FAINTING	
INAPPROPRIATE EMOTIONAL RESPONSE		ALTERTED ALERTNESS		INCREASED ALCOHOL OR DRUG USE		NAUSEA	
GUILT / SHAME		BLAMING/SHAMING		CHANGE IN SEXUAL BEHAVIOR +/-		GRINDING TEETH	
GRIEF		CONFUSION		EMOTIONAL OUTBURSTS		BODY PAIN / HEADACHES	
DENIAL		INTRUSIVE IMAGERY		RESTLESSNESS / UNABLE TO SETTLE		PROFUSE SWEATING	
IRRITABILITY		NIGHTMARES		PACING		CHILLS	
FEAR		POOR ATTENTIVENESS		SUSPICIOUSNESS		MUSCLE TREMORS	
AGITATION		LOW CONCENTRATION		SOCIAL WITHDRAWAL		TWITCHES	
DEPRESSION		DIFFERENT RECALL FROM OTHERS THAT WERE PRESENT		DISINTEREST IN THINGS YOU ONCE ENJOYED		BODY FATIGUE / WEAKNESS	

STRESS COPING QUIZ © GOINGBEYONDTHECALL.LLC		Yes
1	I tend to feel overwhelmed with all there is to do; there is not enough time each day. I no longer feel I have time for the people and experiences I once enjoyed.	
2	I tend to feel like I'm in overdrive and talk, eat, drive, and move around quickly.	
3	I tend to procrastinate or ignore problems wishing they would disappear	
4	I am a workaholic and have difficulty leaving work issues behind, so bring them home with me.	
5	I find it challenging or guilt-inducing to shut down, do nothing or otherwise relax	
6	My mind never stops. Problems and issues take prominence in my brain, and I have trouble concentrating on the things I need to focus on.	
7	Even when I do have appropriate hours of sleep, I wake up tired, fatigued like I haven't slept well.	
8	I am moodier than usual and find my memory is failing me at times.	
9	I tend to speed up slow people up by finishing their sentences or cutting them off.	
10	I tend to be judgmental or critical of other people and find it difficult to offer compliments.	
11	I find it challenging to pay attention when others are speaking. I get lost in my thoughts.	
12	Life is constantly bombarding me with new, and it is hard to finish things or stay on task.	
13	I have aches and pains in my neck, shoulders and back from being tensed up all the time.	
14	No one can do the job to my liking. I prefer to do it myself and don't have the patience to teach.	
15	I tend to be highly competitive and seek to win in most areas and feel frustrated when I don't.	
16	I am easily annoyed and frustrated but don't voice my concerns. I want to avoid any more grief.	
17	My interest in food is changing. Either by eating/bingeing more than usual, or with a loss in appetite.	
18	I have a lot less patience with waiting for anything these days and get easily irritated when impatient.	
19	My dentist or partner has stated I grind my teeth in my sleep.	
20	I have an issue with self-praise and often put myself down or beat myself up over things.	
21	I tend to depend on caffeine, nicotine, alcohol, or drugs to get me through the day and relax me to sleep.	
22	I have less interest in things that once excited me, interests, people, hobbies, even sex.	
23	I have an unhealthy behavior change in gambling, porn, high-risk pursuits, shopping, internet use, or gaming.	
24	I increasingly zone-out, shut people out of my life, and isolate whenever possible.	
	ADD UP YOUR YES ANSWERS	

0-5 points: *You are experiencing normal fluctuations in stress and do not need to be concerned.*

6 – 14 points: *You are moving towards toxic stress levels and need to pay attention to your mental fitness. You are beginning to impact physical, psychological, and relationship health. Build-in daily selfcare routines and be mindful of your communication tactics.*

14 - + points: *You have achieved a damaging level of stress. You are also more likely to experience stress-related illness e.g., diabetes, irritable bowel, migraine, back and neck pain, high blood pressure, heart disease/strokes, mental ill-health (depression, anxiety & PTSD) and unhealthy coping behaviors. Consider professional help to mitigate and reverse the impacts.*

Some stress is good, and we all experience highs and lows when it comes to feeling the stress and pressure to get things done and achieve what's important to us. Where we need to pay attention is when high levels of stress impact our quality of life and relationships. Our brain feeds us what we focus on and when we start spinning in negative stress cycles, we often do not see the damaging influences on our body, mind, and with those we care about until it is at toxic levels. When we fail to cope well with cumulative stress, other body systems start to fail us, and we move into more severe stress-induced diseases and mental health challenges.

MANAGING OUR THINKING - ADAPTIVE RESILIENCY

(Based on Chapters 13 through 20)

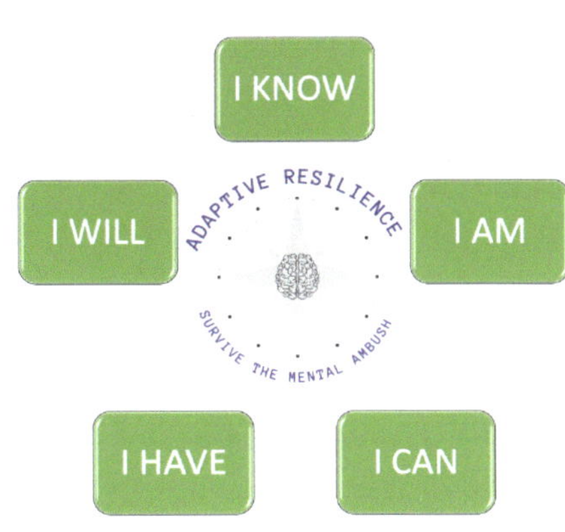

Many public safety professionals start the job with tremendous resiliency. However, the toll on their brain health, nervous system, and long- term physical health is massive. Organizational risk analysis and policy would be very well served to make resiliency building and mental fitness a core training item.

At ***Going Beyond the Call***, we call it "Mental Fitness" for a reason. Like our muscles and our intellect, if we do not exercise them our strength fades. By the end of this program, you will have added many tools to your resiliency toolbox. Our Adaptive Resilience workbook is comprised of five components being:

- 'I know' (psychological injury awareness, prevention, mitigation, understanding)
- 'I am' (inner strengths, resiliency building, and emotional intelligence)
- 'I can' (adaptive coping tools, communication tactics, and wellness strategies)
- 'I have' (peer training, external supports, and building strong connections)
- 'I will' (commit to trauma-informed care approach to optimum mental fitness)

One way to gain command of our brain health is to c-reate a development plan for our adaptive resilience and coping choices. Then to practice them until habits are born, which take around 12 weeks to lock in.

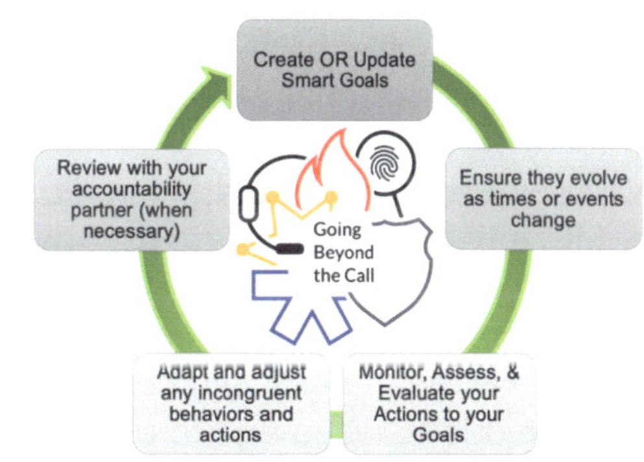

S.M.A.R.T. goals, first utilized in leadership by George T. Doran, is the best formula to create specific, measurable goals that are well thought out and attainable. When goals are developed this way, they are more apt to be realistic and when time is added progress can be tracked. SMART goals are most effective when used as an ***ongoing*** accountability tool. Even better, share them with those you love for shared accountability.

Specific	
Measurable	
Attainable	
Realistic	
Time specific	

What would be your first SMART goal to tackle?

____

____

____

____

MANAGING OUR THINKING – BIAS BUSTING

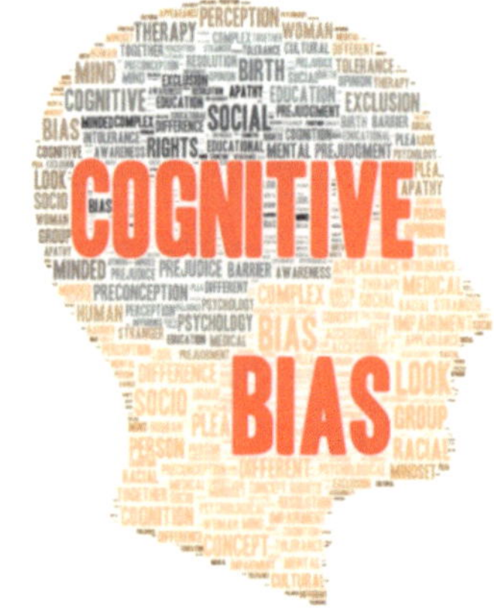

(Bonus briefing from Going Beyond the Call's Bias busting program. Bias training is best served in an interactive environment. This section is not included in our current book but included in our custom design workshops when requested) **For basics watch Implicit Bias | Concepts Unwrapped, youtu.be/OoBvzl-YZf4**

Until we can have difficult conversations about sensitive topics, we will generally fail to truly embrace the mindful management required to rid ourselves of biases that do not serve us, or our society well. The following serves as a brief overview of the broader concept of biased thinking.

The unwanted truth is having bias is not the exception to the rule. We all have them. Our brains need to seek out ways to save energy and time when filtering information to feed our conscious knowledge. They are ingrained in the habits and shortcuts of human cognition.

We will dig deeper into controlling our automated thinking process. With that, we need to grow our awareness to implicit social cognition knowing our brains are wired to filter information with predetermined data. Our subconscious has a deep layer of implicit bias that creeps into our reactivity, often unknowingly, until challenged. Implicit bias is where our response to initial profiling, stereotypes and other cultural, or social differences affect our perceptions, actions, and decision making unconsciously.

Still unsure if you have any biased thinking? You may wish to check yourself with this confidential and free online quiz on many common and currently high-lighted biases. "Project Implicit is a non-profit organization and international collaboration between researchers who are interested in implicit social cognition - thoughts and feelings outside of conscious awareness and control. The goal of the organization is to educate the public about hidden biases and to provide a virtual laboratory for collecting internet data.
https://implicit.harvard.edu/implicit/takeatest.html

What did you learn about yourself? What are some of my known biases? Have you found a difference between your self-projections to others, your explicit bias, and your implicit bias? Does it incentivize you to challenge your biased thoughts? How will you check yourself?

When has new information been accepted and changed the way I feel about something that previously fell outside my comfort zone of cultural, social, and familiar thinking?

____

____

____

Bias is part of the program that our intake and filtering system, the reticular activating system (RAS), uses to scan for threats, unknowns, and things important to us. It is also on the look-out for novel and new things. When we are unaware, ignorant, or conditioned towards things that are different from us or of a different perspective than us, a bias is formed. When we start to investigate these automatic thoughts that pervasively impact our attitudes and actions, we can learn to challenge this deeply imbedded data and pivot to new ways of thinking.

What is fed to our conscious thinking is not intentional. When conscious thought is involved, it is an explicit bias. We know it's there and we chose to show it or hide it. An implicit bias would be involuntarily served up without cognitive processing. It's why we may laugh at a stereotype and then catch ourselves once the look and body language around us hint it is inappropriate. Then we can self-shame, wondering why we had that response when our self-perception believes we are not "racist," "judgmental about others," or "mean."

When we have explicit bias, we know we think about certain things that may be perceived as socially unacceptable and we choose to "pick our audience," or conceal such thoughts for the sake of political correctness. So, we may see ourselves from an overtly declared belief system and still have some actions, word choices, and stances that are contrary to our outward self-projection.

Where has implicit bias conflicted with a public stance you have taken on a bias topic?

____

____

____

MANAGING OUR THINKING - WHY DO WE HAVE BIAS?

Broader bias can also be activated by personalities, behaviors, auto-responsiveness, and actions (more on emotional reactivity in our Ego State section). This is where some of us may 'hide' from our bias thinking. "It wasn't about the color of his skin, it was the way he approached me, or spoke to me." Implicit social contagion creates automated thoughts about other people that are the cause of derogatory attitudes about issues around race, age, sexuality, ethnicity, appearance, and abilities. These biases are programmed early in life and are often deepened due to the social and culture environment you grew up in. We tend to relate best with those like us and so draw into our tribe like-minded folks.

Bias can cross into each general category. Race bias is much broader and deeper than color or ethnic origin. It can be broken down into cultural groups, caste systems, religion, regional territory, and other sub-categories.

It isn't all from childhood either, our social and career circles have great influence over how we 'group' and 'profile' others. In today's social media frenzy this social contagion is greatly impacted by the types of messaging you tune into (more on that coming up). So even when you believe yourself to be unbiased, listen close enough and you will find biased thoughts creep in and show in your behaviors and actions.

Where has implicit social contagion pervasively entered at your workplace, family functions, or your media feeds? Does it seem like you when it comes out, or does it catch you off-guard?

____

____

____

____

____

____

So why does our brain act this way? It is a mental shortcut that allows people to make decisions quickly by bringing their emotional response into play. They make decisions according to their gut feeling. Our brains absorb a tremendous amount of new information every minute. Some of this information we consciously manage, question, work on, mull over and attempt to solve. However, the conscious part of our brain has a limited capacity and to make matters more complicated, we often must think and act quickly.

To help us, our brains use shortcuts that science calls heuristics. Although often incredibly useful and accurate, these internal programs are not perfect and can be impaired with old, outdated, and incorrect information. When our heuristics fail to provide a correct, or helpful insight, the result is cognitive bias. This can lead us to a prejudiced or skewed conclusion without all the relevant and current facts. Consider how very apparent this becomes in US vs THEM scenarios. The emotional distance often drives a wedge into reasoned and collaborative bridge building.

After this section, and the test taken, what unconscious bias should I retire as I retrain my brain to consider a new way of thinking?

____

____

____

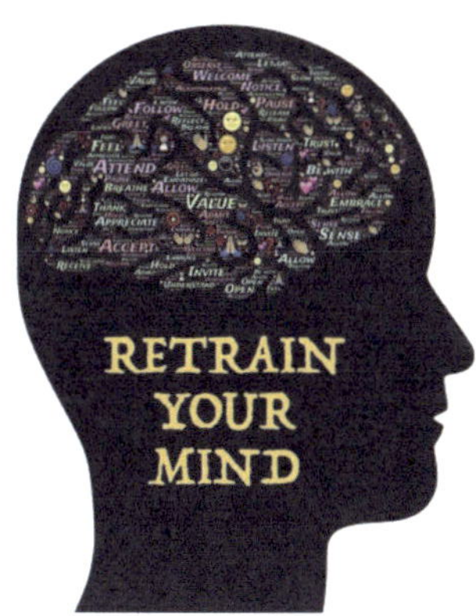

MANAGING OUR THINKING - COMMON COGNITIVE BIASES

The good news is our brains are quite trainable with foundational knowledge and a willingness to challenge, change and evolve unhelpful and hurtful thinking patterns.

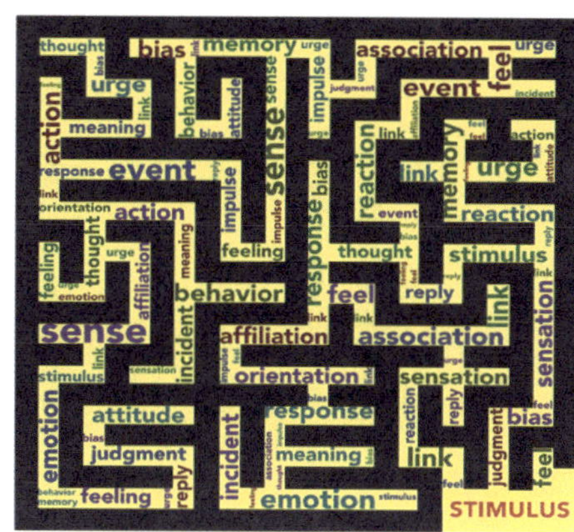

COMMON CONGNITIVE BIASES AND THEIR OVERALL STRUCTURE

A Cognitive Bias Cheat Sheet was created by Buster Benson who went through the 175 known cognitive biases and grouped them by their functions in 20 unique categories. He further identified four general problems that biases help us solve so we can better explore the roots of where our own come from. I like how he states, "Cognitive biases are just tools, useful in the right contexts, harmful in others," as it paves the way to understanding the applied psychology insight that not all cognitive biases are wrong or bad to pay attention to. It would help us all if we learned in school to have a good working knowledge of them when interacting with people and maneuvering through life. Benson identified four major problem clusters. Each of these overall descriptors breaks down further into 180+ known cognitive biases. The full codex is on the next page and hard to read but go online and you can expand each section. The Codex are grouped into categories and rendered by John Manoogian III as a radial dendrogram (circle diagram).

What Should we Remember?	Need to Act Fast	Too Much Information	Not Enough Meaning
We store memories based on HOW they were experienced, and the emotion attached. We reduce events & lists to their key elements We discard specifics under generalities We edit and reinforce emotional memories after the fact	We favor simple options and avoid ambiguous or complex options To avoid mistakes, we aim to preserve autonomy and group status while avoiding irreversible decisions To stay focused, we favor the immediate, relatable thing in front of us	We notice things already primed by memory or repetitiveness Bizarre, funny, & visually striking things stick in our memory strongest We notice when something has changed We are drawn to details that confirm our own existing belief We notice flaws in others MUCH easier than we see flaws in ourselves	We tend to accept stories and patterns even without supporting data We fill in characteristics with stereotypes, generalities, prior history, and cultural programming We imagine things and people we are familiar with or fond of with higher regard We think we know what other people are thinking We project our current mindset & assumptions onto the future and past

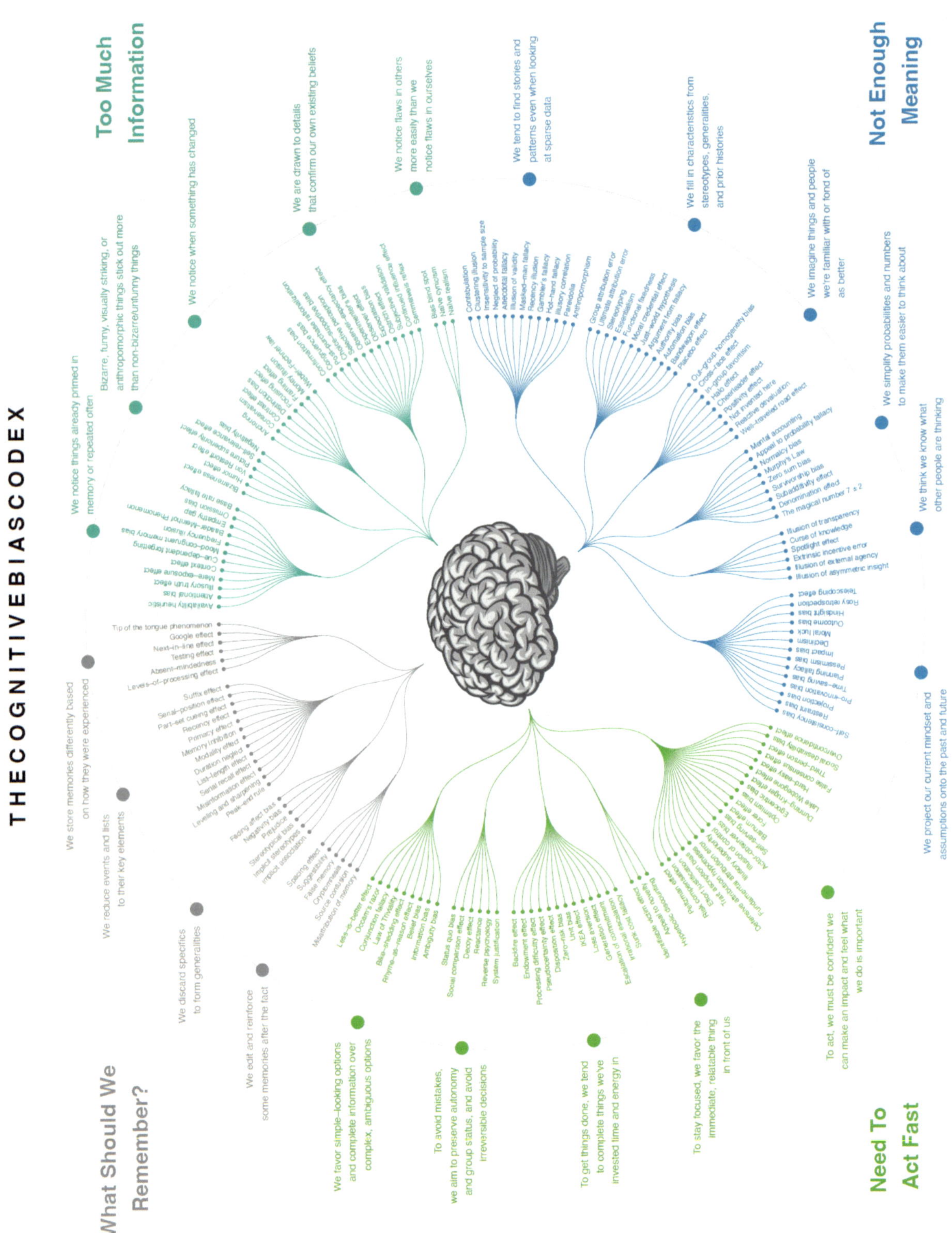

CLICK: Wikipedia link for close up view of codex or search Wikipedia BIAS CODEX

MANAGING OUR THINKING - WHY ARE WE STUBBORN ABOUT OUR BIAS?

Confirmation Bias: Your Brain is So Judgmental

Watch YouTube: https://youtu.be/Blv9054dBBI and https://youtu.be/tZvDaPBqAyg and https://youtu.be/B8ofWFx525s

READ: https://www.scientificamerican.com/article/biases-make-people-vulnerable-to-misinformation-spread-by-social-media/

Implicit Confirmation Bias is the hidden gatekeeper that drives click bait and filters as well as biased and one-sided content to individual social media users. It is influenced by bot-using algorithms that produce filter bubbles. Users of social media platforms are more susceptible to this implicit confirmation bias and more often exposed to misleading, power driven and biased information. The leading algorithms push a tendency to search further, accept opinion assertion, interpret fake intent to opposing opinion in a manner that validates one's pre-existing hypotheses and beliefs.

Without consciously seeking out a balanced perspective confirmation bias can drive our implicit and explicit bias to a socially splitting mindset. It allows us to dehumanize those opposed to our way of thinking.

Confirmation Bias

I have heard from both sides … time to do some research

Internet search until you find your own opinion mirrored

Bingo! I was right! Literally the first link that agrees with what you already believe.

Explicit Confirmation Bias or Desire to confirm our opinions: Once we form an opinion, we typically seek out information that supports it and we ignore facts that challenge it. ***What is an example of this in your world?***

How have internet bots driven your viewing on social media, general news, shopping, and other online experiences? Have you given much thought to the information you are NOT receiving to develop a balanced and thought-provoking perspective?

MANAGING OUR THINKING - COGNITIVE DISTORTION

The public safety professional's life has regular ups and downs with stress and increased negative situations. Regardless of these events and experiences we have the power to choose our attitude internally and outwardly toward others. To combat the mental ambush of repeated stress we must utilize awareness, prevention, and mitigation tactics to challenge why we think the way we do. Then we must question regularly whether these thinking patterns are still working for us? Psychologists describe cognitive distortion as the irrational, inflated beliefs and thoughts that alter one's perception of reality, typically in a negative or harmful way. Although common, most of us are not aware of what to look for as they are subconscious, habitual, automated inputs. Many of us are also unfamiliar with how much power we have to re-program our brains and change what no longer serves our wellness and interactive success. This is an important skillset because cognitive distortions lead to increased depression, anxiety, and stress reactions.

COMMON COGINITIVE DISTORATIONS

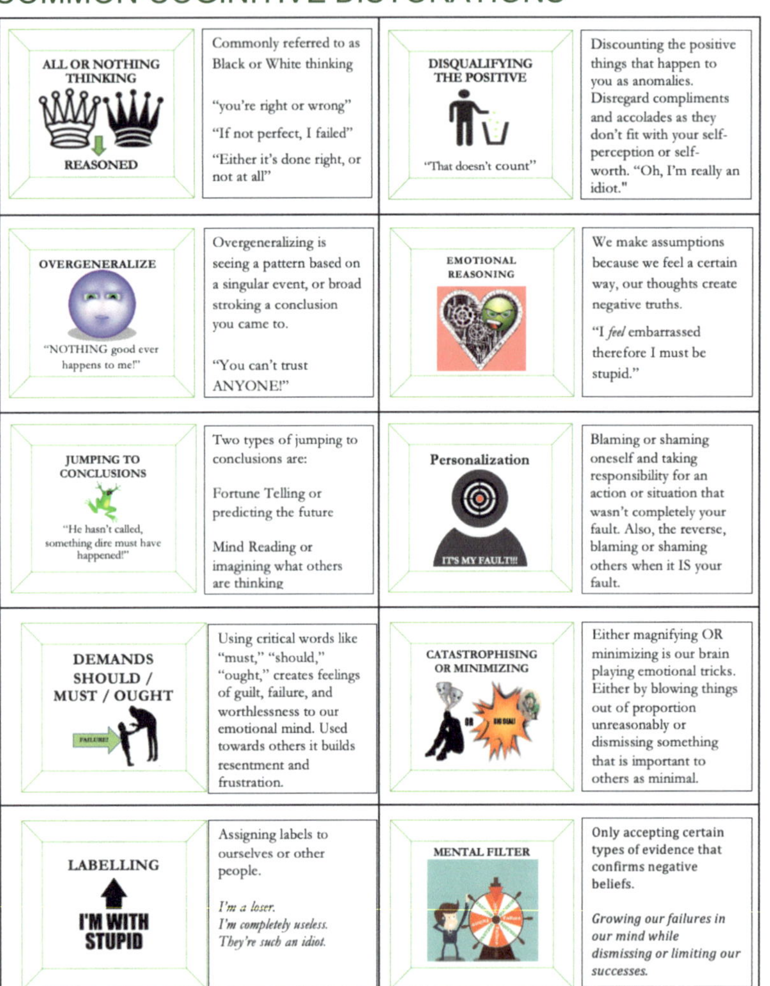

Explore what's stressing you and challenge cognitive distortion by:

- Embracing the positives and benefits
- Figuring out what you CAN change, or control
- Creating 'Lessons Learned' to adapt or change for the next time
- Growing perspective by creating a list of positive vs. negative
- Get the facts vs. guessing– clarify your mind reading ways if you don't know for sure
- Asking what you know to be the absolute truth
- Challenging should/never/always statements
- Removing negative labels from self-talk
- Expanding responsibility to the known / unknown

More Cognitive worksheets are available at psychologytools.com

Choose one of your Cognitive Distortions. How will you challenge your thinking now?

____

____

MANAGING OUR THINKING - EMOTIONAL COMPREHENSION

The emotion wheel created after years of studying and research by American psychologist Dr. Robert Plutchik. He proposed we have eight primary emotions that are the foundation for all others. These emotions are joy, sadness, acceptance, disgust, fear, anger, surprise, and anticipation. His book, ***Emotions and Life: Perspectives from Psychology, Biology, and Evolution,*** delves into identifying our emotions and how to act accordingly. He is quoted as saying, *"Once we objectify and understand the emotions, we can empathize with ourselves, and channel our focus in the direction of emotions we actually want to feel."*

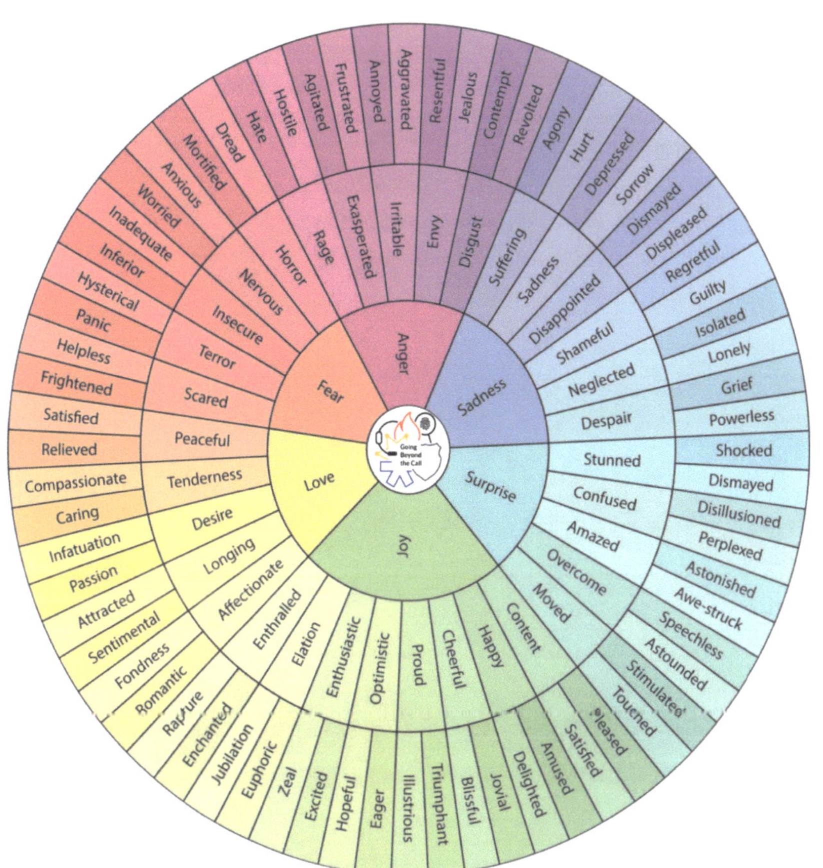

There isn't much education on emotional intelligence (more on that later) nor how to express our emotions well. Would it surprise you to learn there are around 34,000 identified emotions? That we typically feel the spread of a couple of thousand emotions daily: 3-5 emotions in a minute. (Marc Brackett, EI Superpowers studies)

If the human experience is meant to be expressed with such variety, shouldn't we know more about how to aptly identify how we feel about something? Give yourself permission to feel and you may just be surprised at the increased self-control when you need it.

DEVELOPING OUR FEELINGS DESCRIPTORS – Think of a scenario that evokes emotion. What is the feeling? Using the emotion wheel describe it fully. Where does it come from?

____

____

____

____

____

____

MANAGING OUR THINKING - EMOTIONAL SPIRIALING

Why is being mindful of how you are feeling and being able to aptly describe it beneficial to trauma-informed maturity? Our brains need to process the unimaginable things dealt with shift to shift. When something is disturbing enough to cause a traumatic stress injury, understanding how to describe it properly in our heads will help the process of settling the event into memory. When we cannot process these experiences well, the spinning or continuous replay may occur. Repeated playback, nightmares, sleeplessness, intrusive thoughts can move a traumatic stress injury into a PTSD diagnosis.

When it comes to self-care, you want to be able to dig a little deeper into the mood, behavior, or reactivity you experience to evaluate whether it's serving your wellness and the relationships that matter most to you. You want to deploy the tactics and tools you are learning here to move you out of an unhealthy mental ambush. With practiced skill, you are less likely to respond to your next call with the remnants of trauma reaction simmering in your brain and showing in your body language. Being mindful and utilizing grounding exercises allows us more cognitive control over our emotional reactivity. With unconscious competence, it enables us to shift or re-frame the emotional spiraling that can do us harm and change our state immediately.

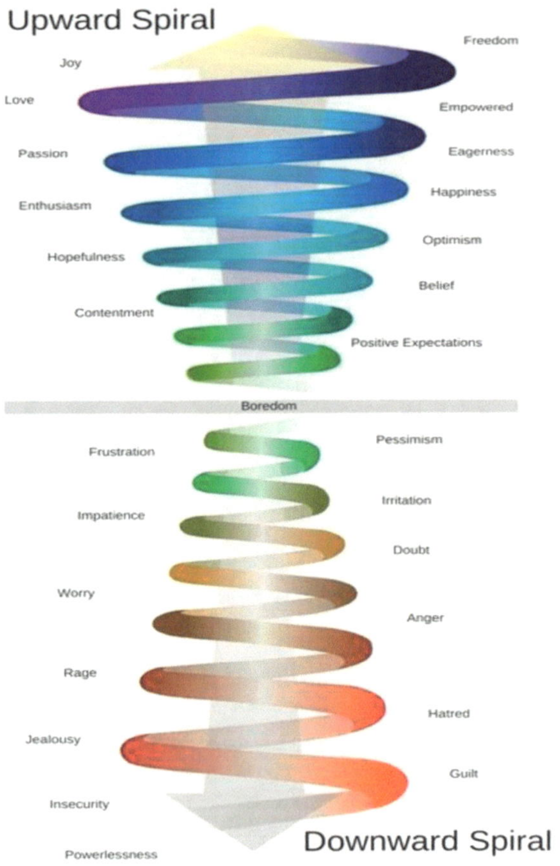

Abraham-Hicks Emotional Guidance Scale can aid moving ourselves from one emotional level to another.
The goal is to use mindful and cognitive exercises to move up one level at a time. With controlled effort to change our state, we manifest the emotions that serve us best. Have you ever met someone that changes the 'mood' of a room just by entering? We all emit an energy that can be felt by others; it can calm, or it can negatively escalate those we interact with before we say one word. By managing our emotional reactivity, we can better manage our interactions and influence others. Control your emotions, don't let your emotions control you!

What is your key take-away on how your energy, mood and emotional state impacts the emotional reactivity of those you interact with?

____

____

MANAGING OUR THINKING: COGNITIVE BEHAVIOR TOOLS

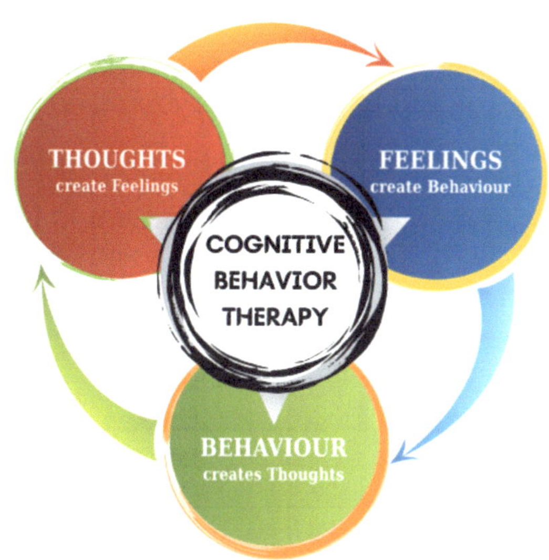

COGNITIVE BEHAVIOR THERAPY (CBT) is commonly used to aid stress, anxiety, depression and other "thought hijacking" brain patterns to provide corrective emotional experiences. CBT works through the connectivity and relationships between thoughts, feelings, actions, and the body or physiological reactions.

The focus intersects four environmental areas that summarize our past (relationships, family, ACE's, with both life turmoil and success in our current state. This includes our root support systems (as discussed earlier in this workbook) and current social/emotional challenges, career, environmental, and societal influences.

Think of a self-defeating thought that goes through your mind regularly. Consider the potential ways to re-evaluate this thought using this thinking process chart. How does moving the thought around change your view?

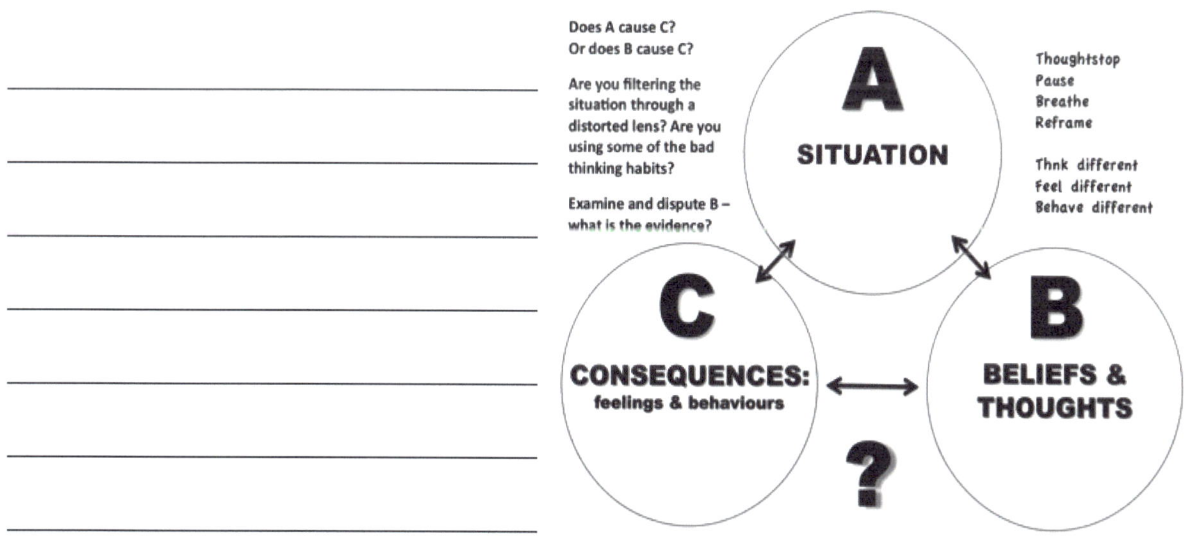

All of our tactics and tips on managing your brain helps self-care awareness, prevention, mitigation, and action tactics to manage the guaranteed stress of the job. If you still aren't convinced a little self-assessment and work would be helpful, lets jump to the next two worksheets where we can put our investigative hats on and question the logic of our thinking patterns and wellness choices. After which we will delve into the trauma responses that may need support or professional assistance to help re-set your brain.

EXERCISE: Creating incentive to change:

Investigative Psychology:

Have you ever wanted to put someone on trial? What about YOURSELF? Your irrational thoughts – cognitive distortions – that lead into a pattern of feeling bad about yourself or others?

Use this worksheet to put your thoughts on trial. You can record your cognitive distortions, irrational, and automatic thoughts that are causing you harm. Then drill down and answer with evidence and facts that refute the distorted thought.

The Crime: Describe the upsetting event:

____

____

____

____

____

____

The Victim perspective: What automatic thoughts come to mind about the event?

____

____

____

____

____

The Prosecution perspective: Identify the name of the Cognitive Distortion and a rational response – a more realistic thought that refutes the automatic thoughts.

____

____

____

____

____

EXERCISE: Analyzing reasons for change:

Cost-benefit Analysis:

Use this worksheet to break down the personal cost to benefit outcome for working through an attitude or irrational belief that you would like to change.

The Attitude or Belief I Want to Change:

Advantages of Believing This:

Disadvantages of Believing This:

Benefits and positive outcomes possible by changing this belief:

TRAUMATIC STRESS INJURIES
(Refer to Chapter 3,6,7,8)

This section provides an understanding of traumatic stress reactions, common responses, and suggestions on self-care. Understanding this helps you interact better with the community you serve. It helps you lead your organizational wellness from a command or peer perspective. It allows you to look in the mirror and understand what the heck is going on inside when you must manage the unthinkable shift after shift. Most events you experience will quickly become "just part of the job," however, there will also be those that 'stick' and are harder to shake. Perhaps the victim reminded us of someone or something you witnessed as a youth. Perhaps it was truly unimaginable, and your brain strained to make sense of it. There are many ways an event can grip our inner horror or disbelief.

What was the first scene/event that really shook your senses? What coping mechanism did you use, if any? Who did you share it with?

____

____

____

When we think of psychological trauma we often jump to PTSD. Public safety does not currently have consistent statistics, but the research shows that a range of 10 – 19% across disciplines will be diagnosed with this disorder. The broader health impact is not nearly as recognized. Everyone, and I mean, EVERYONE, experiences the general wear and tear of these high stress roles though. Most wellness training and agency focus is on the "after effect" of psychological injury or the risk and liability requirements. Which means they tend to utilize de-escalation training over preventative efforts and wellness programs, and many will offer critical incident stress debriefings after a crisis or highly disturbing incident. These remain good strategies and important tools on the toolbelt of every staff.

Have critical incident stress debriefings helped you overcome the long-term effects of a really bad call? What do you wish could have been added to help you manage the experience?

____

____

____

It is not that great help options are not available, there are so many to choose from. However, the timing of most choices miss a huge opportunity to get ahead of many psychological injury situations by preparing individuals for the mental ambush. As example, even those created for the sole benefit of the member, like the majority of chaplain, peer support solutions, and employee assistance programs, focus on the aftermath, when worst moment has passed. Either after the traumatic event, or after the outcome of behavior, safety, or relationship stress puts someone's livelihood and wellness at risk. There are many great non-profit and external support services to help with suicide prevention, and with supports that can also aid PTSD, *IF* the person suffering has enough awareness to recognize and seek help.

Post event management simply misses the preventative risk mark when it comes to proactive efforts. There is drain on both the budget and harmful long term health outcomes that isn't typically measured. For most of the highly resilient staff in these professions it isn't the major event that will do them in, it is the nagging, persistent drain on their mind and body that costs them good health, relationships, and strong mental fitness. Many do not even have the awareness to recognize the slow slip into maladaptive actions and behaviors that burden one's mind and body throughout a career and into retirement. It costs the agency in safety issues, performance investigations, lawsuits, and increasing short/long term disability costs. When it comes to retention and recruitment, staff want to know that administration has their back and will protect their health with preventative measures show that commitment. Without strong preventative minded leadership this easy proactive fix is not typically on administrations radar.

Many disparaging remarks from line personnel are on the lack of care from leadership and administration so ***Going Beyond the Call's Prepare for the Mental Ambush*** is focused on repairing and improving this gap in employee engagement and budget intelligence. Further, most internal investigations on conduct unbecoming do not have a trauma-informed approach which fails to recognize the underlying causes of the situation. Mandatory psychological evaluations *after* a major incident or on an annual basis are great and if leadership prioritized a trauma-informed care approach to self-care it would be measurably better. This is where we come in strong; preparing for the mental ambush gives each member the awareness and tactics to grow their adaptive resilience and prevent and mitigate many stressful and traumatic moments. It also provides the knowledge and removes the stigma of activating further support and services when self-care is not meeting their mental fitness needs.

At ***Going Beyond the Call*** our approach of trauma-informed pre-escalation changes potentially negative outcomes, reducing risk and liability challenges. We believe a culture shift of how organizations view their fiscal and human resource investment can save many minds from very dark places. Preparing for the mental ambush on inevitable ambush of events, experiences, and effects from traumatic exposure will avoid the personal, professional, and public cost currently managed after the fact. Will it help these worst-case outcomes? Absolutely! Will it avoid the 34% of members who are diagnosed burnout, depression, compassion fatigue? You bet it will. This cultural shift in exposing the root cause of many risk and liability issues in these professions directly effects the mental fitness of members, their service to communities, and it drastically impacts budgets and bottom-line results.

Research on the cognitive processing and limbic system impairment through brain imaging and neuroscience studies indicate different backgrounds, resiliency thresholds, experiences and support systems impact these professions in several ways.

Have you ever attended to an event and had a completely different experience and post-event recall than your co-workers? Did you believe it to be normal for you, or them, to feel differently?

____

____

DIRECT & INDIRECT TRAUMA - AND COMBATING THAT 'ONE' THING THAT REALLY GETS TO YOU...

"There isn't a timestamp for psychological trauma injury; many do not feel the impacts of stress injuries until after retirement. They bottle it up until there's nothing else to think about. Others survived so much they think they are immune until 'one thing' pops open their emotional vault and turns their life upside down. Preparing for the mental ambush, at any stage of your career is the key for long term wellness and quality of life."
~ Deirdre von Krauskopf

The Diagnostic and Statistical Manual of Mental Disorders IV-TR (American Psychiatric Association [APA], 2000) defines trauma as *"Direct personal experience of an event that involves actual or threatened death or serious injury, or other threat to one's physical integrity; or witnessing an event that involves death, injury, or a threat to the physical integrity of another person; or learning about unexpected or violent death, serious harm, or threat of death or injury experienced by a family member or other close associate."*

Typically, those exposed to psychological trauma shows some signs and symptoms as defined in our previous stress section. Natural human responses to unnatural events will cause notable spikes outside our window of tolerance. Generally, the professionals in the field of psychology agree that the signs of trauma can spike to an Acute Stress Disorder, or another emerging term, Post Traumatic Stress Injury. It is generally believed you have approximately 12 weeks before this level of untreated or unmanaged stress injury can be diagnosed as PTSD.

This is the window of response time to be utilizing the self-care tactics in this program. When self-management is failing to calm the internal turmoil, knowing this window of time is incentive to ask for other forms of mental first aid treatment. For organizations this is the window where peer-to-peer, critical incident stress management interventions, chaplains, or psychologists can aid PTSD avoidance. Notable though, is research indicating those who naturally default to hypo-arousal (shutting down/avoidance indicators) may be further triggered by CISM programs. Every person is different, so organizations should ensure training, like ours, prepares them for all the variations of trauma reactions and how to move through their default nervous system response. What we regularly hear in our workshops is that there are so many disturbing moments that just don't rate a CIT response. So even when organizations have options, many don't understand when to reach out for help.

To move from heightened stress reactions to traumatic stress injury one's affected response to the event must involve intense fear, helplessness, or horror (for children, the affected response involves disorganized or agitated behavior). Generally direct and indirect is differentiated by:

Direct = personal involvement in a traumatic event

Indirect = witnessing a traumatic event or exposure to trauma (this also includes secondary or vicarious trauma as often felt by communications, forensics, corrections, and even families)

Think of a couple of events that really got to you. Identify one that was direct, and another that was indirect?

DIRECT	INDIRECT

There isn't much data on public safety exposure to indirect trauma. Researchers, Zimring, Gulliver, Knight, Munroe, & Keane (2006) briefly studied direct and indirect trauma exposure for 9/11. They identified direct exposure as either experiencing or witnessing the event. While indirect exposure was defined as becoming aware of highly disturbing news, such as unexpected or violent death of a family member. They concluded that PTSD may be developed from indirect exposure to trauma.

Many in public safety feel a brotherhood or sisterhood at work, so they are deeply impacted by members' death and injury, even outside their agency. From this researched opinion we can start to understand how many in the public safety realm, who are regularly and repeatedly exposed to indirect trauma, develop psychological, physiological, and behavioral challenges. It didn't happen *TO* them, but they were very much part of the event and experience and therefore may suffer incident based and cumulative trauma effects. For others, they bury it down repeatedly until the vault bursts open after that 'one more thing' triggers the brain's inability to cope any further. All these paths lead to maladaptive coping and extreme stress responses like addictions, 'behavior unbecoming' scenarios, relationship breakdowns, mental or physical disorders, up to and including PTSD and suicidality.

We don't often think about that 'one thing.' Consider a time when a call was like dozens you have been to before but this one hit hard. Jot down why you believe this event pushed open the vault?

____

____

____

____

The mental health aspect is one concern, and another is the physiological impact (administrators and risk managers take note). There is direct correlation between psychological trauma and physical health conditions such as diabetes, chronic obstructive pulmonary disease (COPD), heart disease, cancer, and high blood pressure (what are the employee stats on these?).

Even the most resilient, the ones who claim they can compartmentalize and lock it away, fall prey to the long term (often post retirement) impacts of a career with repeated stress injuries. Left unmanaged, these professionals also experience lower life spans. With proper prevention and mitigation, we can change these known outcomes.

In the military, soldiers are taught to prepare for the ambush both mentally and physically. They are exposed under numerous scenarios to act and react to ambushes. We do not build the mental fitness of our public safety personnel the same way. Even knowing, without any doubt, that members will be psychologically ambushed several times throughout their career and suffer physically over the long term. Add on our ability to lessen the tragic statistics for suicides among the ranks and the need to act now becomes clear. Programs like, ***Going Beyond the Call ~ Prepare for the Mental Ambush***, should become CORE training mandates.

Most entering these professions start their careers with higher-than-average resiliency. Even knowing this, the impact on the brain and nervous system after repeated direct, indirect, and cumulative trauma is not well studied until it morphs into a full-blown disorder such as depression or PTSD. We urge you all to take control of your mental fitness NOW. It can make a world of difference to your mental, physical and relationship health.

"Preparation leads to preservation ~ Procrastination leads to devastation."
~ Sean Wyman

How has this section's insight changed how I view traumatic stress injuries for myself, my peers, and my profession? Journaling as you go is a great way for the mind to assimilate the lessons into a reality check for future resiliency growth.

STRESS INJURY RESPONSE LOOKS LIKE:

How many of these are familiar to you, now or in the past?					
	Sudden sweating		Emotional exhaustion		Nightmares or flashbacks
	Heart palpitations		Fear, Anxiety, Depression		Easily startled
	More suspectable to colds/flu, illnesses, post major events		Headaches / Stomachaches / Backaches		Constipation or diarrhea
	Spiked increase in sex (affairs, casual sex) or disinterest/inability to arouse		Increased use of alcohol / drugs / overeating		Outbursts of rage or anger Easily agitated over things that never used to get to you
	Emotional swings (family is walking on eggshells)		Sudden changes to sleep quality (too much/little)		Desire to isolate oneself or feeling detached
	Difficulty trusting others / feelings of betrayal		Self-blame, survivors' guilt, or shame (didn't make the save, wasn't there in time)		Diminished interest in everyday activities

SECONDARY TRAUMA

SECONDARY TRAUMATIC STRESS (STS) is associated with every public safety professional's job. Every bad call, grieving human, hopeless moment, horrifying incident builds up in cumulative stress and trauma. Not only events you directly participated in, but from other members or calls in your agency. It also comes home with you even when you try to hide it. This area is where some family members may also be affected when they worry or stress about your safety and how your job impacts or changes you. Getting them involved by sharing this work will enhance their mental fitness and will help build connections and understanding of the stress you bring home from your shifts. Creating accountability agreements to manage stress will bring families closer together.

Secondary Trauma shows as:

Fear in situations that others would not think were frightening	Wary of every situation, expecting a traumatic outcome	Easily startled, feeling "jumpy" or "on guard" all of the time
A feeling of responsibility or a strong belief that others' trauma is yours	Feeling powerless, or excessively worrying that something terrible will happen to you, loved ones or colleagues	Sense of being haunted by the troubles you see and hear from others

Have you seen these symptoms in yourself, in a peer, or in a loved one?

____

____

____

Several studies show that psychological stress reverberates beyond the person who is experiencing the direct or even indirect trauma. The extent of the emotional, behavioral, and nervous system response can impact shift partners, family, friends and your significant other. This trauma has a few sub-categories: vicarious trauma; compassion fatigue; burnout; and hypervigilance (one of the PTSD symptoms) which we will address in the coming pages.

Studies in PTSD and trauma victims show there are often negative impacts to relationship satisfaction. This includes avoidance or decreased emotional intimacy, less sexual activity, loss of friendship intimacy, increased frustration and argumentativeness, and less communication connectivity between couples. Not surprising then, that the direct, indirect, and cumulative trauma events experienced by public safety professionals lead to higher separation and divorce rates. A consistent effort in building mental fitness can change that, especially when you bring your significant other into the learning experience. As a support person, or as an accountability partner, I can tell you from personal experience, when you are involved, things fare much better than when you are shut out.

There is a loneliness, and for some, the grief felt by partners watching their loved one turn into an entirely different person. In Deirdre's program, "***Behind the Badge ~ The Home Effect of Serve and Protect,***" she coined the term *'PTSD Widow'* due to the deep sense of loss for the loved one that is no longer there. She received vigorous nods and expressions of agreement from many spouses who experienced the same feeling. Without good relationship communication and connected mental fitness neither partner has the knowledge, or patience, needed to work through the trauma impacts of 'the job'. Loss of intimacy can also occur and lead to spiraling thoughts that the partner is cheating, impacting trust, even when unfounded. Trying to find a logical reason why things are falling apart may lead the brain on a hurtful and unnecessary journey. This may compound issues of self-worth and self-esteem within your significant other with feeling like they are not '*enough*'. Not knowing how to save the relationship may lower someone on *Maslow's Hierarchy of Needs* and cause anxiety and distress over their safety and security needs or result in their own unhealthy coping mechanisms manifesting.

Have you ever had challenges in your current or past relationship where you knew it was spiraling negatively but you didn't have the knowledge or mental effort to know how to fix it? Would some of what you have learned thus far helped? In what way? (Just wait for the Communications section!)

____

____

____

____

____

Without both parties seeking supportive answers to manage the broken connectivity and recreate a healthy relationship, saving it can be hard to accomplish. When neither have had any awareness training in mental fitness and have no idea what's happening inside both brains, then seeking that help may not even be on their radar.

If seeking professional counselling, it is very important to find a therapist who has experience working with public safety professionals and who, ideally, practices trauma-informed care treatments. It's also important to note that the first therapist or support option may not resonate with you, and more than one option may need to be explored. Trauma therapy is highly personal and, like any relationship, finding the right fit will go a long way towards success. Like a doctor, dentist, chiropractor, veterinarian, if we don't click well with them, then quit them, but don't stop the healing effort. Your health and wellness are worth looking for that professional help that best suits you and what you want to achieve. You can even ask the therapist by sharing you are not resonating with them and can they recommend someone else. Most will know the styles and personalities of their peers in the area.

Have you ever tried a therapy option and been disappointed? Did you seek someone new or investigate further help?

____

____

____

____

Reaching out for therapeutic help has some other stumbling blocks. There is a noted lack of trust in the public safety community that what they share won't get leaked and adversely affect their career. Most agencies these days allow for benefits to be used across a wide variety of options. If you don't trust the local therapist, or fear running into someone you know coming and going in a small town, then seek support elsewhere, even online.

Some fear the requirement to share due to the 'harm to self or others clause' which obliges a peer support or therapy source to engage a formal mental health check, based on local laws. This can equate a hopeless feeling that one cannot be honest about suicidal, self-harming, or rage issues. If your trust issues are heightened due to this, then a healthy resource can be a local or near town Chaplain (non-denominational), or Minister. They have a unique freedom to dialogue (unless the threat is imminent) about topics such as rage or suicidal thoughts, without the same stringent action requirements. Finding a Chaplain with public safety or military training will greatly aid finding an amazing supportive lifeline dedicated to helping you seek out a path to wellness. If you don't have a Chaplain in your area, contact the Director of First Responder Chaplain Division info@SpiritualCareAssociation.org. ***Going Beyond the Call*** presented to their International Chaplains Association Conference about their own mental fitness. It is an amazing organization dedicated to those that serve, they will find you a local resource.

If you are supporting a peer recognize that some may feel hesitant to share their true feelings and struggles with their significant other because they believe the relationship is already close to the end and any information shared (on maladaptive behaviors, as example), may be used against them should relationship failure or divorce become the outcome. In this case we recommend a trauma informed counselor who is experienced with public safety professions lead this delicate balance of sharing to repair vs harming a relationship that is already too far gone to turn around.

"It's hard to overemphasize the need for self-awareness. When it comes to your overall mental, emotional, relational, spiritual, physical, health. We're very complex beings, so it's never just one facet of our lives that starts to breakdown, or be put on pause, that causes any of us to start to have self-doubt and thoughts of hurting ourselves or suicide. Self-awareness is critical. Preemptively, we must learn to really work at our own health, our own well-being in all of its various facets — spiritually, mentally, emotionally. "When you call a chaplain, it is one-hundred percent confidential. People have had inhibitions because they're worried about their careers and reputations, but unless the person who contacts the chaplain release the chaplain from that obligation, they're forbidden to discuss anything,"
~ Army Chaplain (Lt. Col.) Scott Koeman

Often different types of events will evoke different emotional reactions. When you complete your 'GO-TO' list to call refer to your roots exercise. You may wish to list people according to how they support you in the different dimensions of wellness. Whether a close peer, family, or friend, a Chaplain or local Minister, or even a stranger on the helpline, all are important to list.

List the names and numbers of those you would call in a crisis moment. Chaplains, peer support, hotlines. We offer a selection at the back of our book and workbook if you need it.

EVENT TYPE	GO-TO PERSON	CELL #	BACK UP PERSON	CELL #

At times, doing some self-work and research may help open a dialogue for difficult conversations. A very straight forward online relationship practitioner is John Gottman (Gottman.com) who predicts divorce with 97% accuracy. He teaches a trauma-informed approach to therapists, so if you like his style, you may seek out a local practitioner who has taken his training as further support. This may also help couples before trauma has moved the relationship into the danger zone. **Watch: Making Marriage Work: youtu.be/AKTyPgwfPgg**
Find a therapist: Gottman Referral Network

What is your biggest fear in sharing the internal demons and challenges you struggle with? Do you wish you have a stronger bond with your spouse, family, or friends to work through these issues with support?

____

____

____

Using the Roots exercise completed earlier, build a self-care plan, and commit to exploring different options until you find methods that work best for you. You can break it down into the sections we provided or that you created yourself based on your interests and what calms your mind and body. In your workbook/journal or on your computer create a Self-Care plan:

SELF-CARE PLAN EXAMPLE – FILL IN YOUR OWN ACTION PLAN					
PHYSICAL		MENTAL/PSYCHOLGICAL		SPIRITUAL	
	Prep healthy shift meals		Emotional intelligence		Develop hope/gratitude
	Exercise min. 20/day		Peer/Support Groups		Daily thankful for ....
	Calming brain/body (yoga, tai-chi, meditate)		Learn new skills or develop a healthy habit		Contribute/Volunteer to aid a cause you believe in
	Body reset (massage, chiro, fun activity)		Say no to extra responsibilities		Make time for consistent prayer, meditation
	Planned get away		Get out into nature		Seek inspiration
	Develop healthy love/sex outlet		Self-reflect, journal, talk out your ups and downs		Identify and honor what is meaningful in your life
	Remove yourself from triggers where you can		Identify triggers that flare poor behavior, learn their root cause.		Use mindfulness exercises that calm your mind. Practice until automatic.

VICARIOUS TRAUMA

Vicarious trauma is a cumulative experience as these internal changes begin to impact relationships with self, peers and those who matter most. It often ties closely with compassion fatigue and is often felt by others before being recognized in yourself. Vicarious trauma is less focused on specific trauma symptoms and more on the cumulative exhaustion of exposure to repeated details of others trauma. When peers, friends or family members start to raise concerns about your mannerisms, behavior and attitude changing, pay attention! This is your mental warning sign that more serious mental, physical and relationship ailments are developing.

Vicarious trauma shows as:

Lacking a balanced sense of self. You take on too much, try to control events, have difficulty leaving the job behind, or take the work too personally.	Feelings of professional or relationship inadequacy. Second guessing yourself and feelings of insecurity when previously confident.	Desire to emotionally or physically withdraw from people or situations that trigger difficult thoughts and emotions.
Minimizing and trivializing events with comparison to other more traumatic ones.	Increased anger and cynicism that is increasingly difficult to manage or control.	Diminished concentration and difficulty with decision making.
Inappropriate or unhealthy behaviors growing in work or personal life (addictive tendencies).	Increase in physical, emotional, and spiritual fatigue/exhaustion. Increased aches and pains.	Avoidance behaviors. Pushing others away and coping by shutting down and disconnecting.

Vicarious trauma can happen in spurts. Can you think of a time when these mental check outs occurred?

____

____

What can I do about it?

- Check your mental pulse, take assessments provided or linked in this workbook.
- Increase knowledge and awareness about trauma impacts.
- Push against your comfort level, seek out connection with significant other, positive peers, support groups and friends to balance the negativity.
- Build resilience, be diligent and forceful in your self-care routines.
- Create new routines and hobbies to shake up stale or unhelpful ones.
- Build your lessons learned and gratefulness mindset after every call or stress reaction
- Document and post/share positive calls/experiences, build team acknowledgement for the good calls, sharing a more balanced perspective of the good against the bad
- Where lacking, advocate and create peer support groups and healthy group activities.
- Cultivate friendships from varied backgrounds and careers.
- Feed your brain new experiences moving away from 'job tunnel vision'.

BURNOUT

"A state of physical, emotional and mental exhaustion caused by long-term involvement in emotionally demanding situations" ~ Pines & Aronson, 1988

BURNOUT SHOWS AS:

Physically, mentally & emotionally drained	Feeling of reduced personal accomplishment	Emotional exhaustion – feel all used up
Cynicism – detached from job	Poor work performance	"I don't give a damn"
Angry or hopeless	Apathetic	

BURNOUT creeps up with the persistent presence of chronic stress, spiking outside of the window of tolerance consistently. There are four common indicators to burnout:

- **Cynicism:** Lessening of compassion and engagement to the people they serve and increasing feelings of anger, blame or judgment.
- **Disengagement:** When compassion begins to dissipate, then avoidance of emotional engagement grows, often beyond the public being served. It will start as disengagement, but if left unchecked will often grow into broader avoidance of peers, friends, mentors and eventually family members.
- **Dissatisfaction:** With the job or indifference to the work will become more notable and an increase in beating oneself up and expressing thoughts of hopelessness.
- **Exhaustion:** Burnout goes beyond being tired, it is utter exhaustion but often challenged with insomnia. An increase in stimulant/depressant use, unhealthy food, and other addictive behaviors will become more predominant. Overall, it seems like you are not 'all there,' and effectiveness and safety should become a concern for peers and command.

BURN OUT QUIZ	1 Never	2 At Times	3 Often	4 Always
How often are you tired and lacking energy to go to work?				
How often do you feel physically drained, like your batteries are dead?				
How often is your thinking process sluggish or your concentration impaired?				
How often do you feel emotionally detached from co-workers (or customers) and unable to be sensitive to their needs?				
TOTALS				

Rate yourself on each question then total your points from all four questions.

SCORE: If you scored less than nine, you are not suffering from burnout. If you scored between 10 and 12, you are on the verge of burnout. If you scored between 13 and 16, you are suffering full-on burnout.

MANAGING BURNOUT

Tactics to stop the burnout build up:

Use the power of no, practice self-care	Get proper quality and quantity of sleep
Healthy eating habits & staying hydrated	Exercise routine with sitting exercises if sedentary
Mind/Body connection activities (tai-chi, meditation)	Work with a therapist if life is impacted
Take time to journal - process the ugliness of the job by helping your hippocampus process	Create a work end ritual to help leave work behind (music, workout, book on tape)
Practice your spiritual beliefs or if non spiritual, find quiet reflective time alone	Build your tribe of primarily positive, low drama friends and acquaintances

Which of these managing burnout techniques would work best for you?

FINDING BALANCE – one way to practice self-care is use this tool to prioritize your life. WATCH: How the Eisenhower Matrix can fix your Procrastination issues https://youtu.be/k7xJwo1fVyU

LIST MONTHLY ACTIVITIES	DATE:		DO 1ST	NEXT STEPS *MUST DO *TRACK PROGRESS	DATE:		DEFER & SCHEDULE	NEXT STEPS *PUT IN CALENDER *TRACK PIECES *INVITE OTHERS
	URGENT & IMPORTANT	1				1		
		2				2		
		3				3		
		4				4		
		5				5		
		6				6		
		7				7		
		8				8		
	DATE:		DELEGATE	NEXT STEPS *AUTOMATE *WHO CAN DO	DATE:		DELETE	NEXT STEPS *REMOVE FROM LIFE *MARK FOR LATER
	URGENT & IMPORTANT	1				1		
		2				2		
		3				3		
		4				4		
		5				5		
		6				6		
		7				7		
		8				8		
WHERE DO YOU SPEND MOST OF YOUR TIME? IS IT HELPING GROW YOUR MENTAL FITNESS? DOES IT BRING YOU JOY, FULFILLMENT, ACHIEVEMENT, AND CONTRIBUTE TO YOUR GOALS? @GOINGBEYONDTHECALL.COM								

COMPASSION FATIGUE

Compassion Fatigue is measured differently than other Secondary Traumas. Given those in "helping or serving" roles choose their professions, compassion fatigue must be measured against your overall quality of life and job satisfaction. This area of mental fatigue is about the balance of good and service you provide, against those dark days when your mind cannot cope with what you see, do, touch, smell, hear and respond to. The brain and gut (where most of our serotonin is made) will desperately override any "willpower" to get a fix of feel-good chemicals. Layer on ACE's, where you are on Maslow's Hierarchy of needs and your developed emotional intelligence, and this can be ground zero for addictive behavior.

Take the test Quality of Life Scale (PROQOL), which compares compassion strain with compassion and work satisfaction. proqol.org/uploads/ProQOL_5_English_Self-Score.pdf

COMPASSION FATIGUE SHOWS AS:

Physical signs like a racing heart, shortness of breath, and increased tension headaches	Feeling you are not doing your job well enough, a reduced sense of meaning	Turning to numbing or mind-altering substances (alcohol or drugs) to cope
Anger, Embitterment, Cynicism	Frustration with self, others, or organization	Feeling like a failure, despair
Shattered Assumptions (no good in people/world)	Tired, even exhausted, and often overwhelmed	Disconnected from others, lacking feelings, indifferent
Interpersonal problems and conflict	Helplessness / Hopeless	Apathy and Mistrust
Loss of interest in activities you used to enjoy	Worry about the future	Loss of meaning for your life or life's purpose
Difficulty making decisions	Spiritual/Relational challenges	Decreased self-esteem
Confusion/memory problems	Emotional numbness	Irritable/ hypersensitivity
GI tract problems	Neck/backaches	Anxiety
Sleep problems	Withdrawal, disconnection	Feeling powerless

These professionals have also found that their empathy and ability to connect with their loved ones and friends are impacted by compassion fatigue. In turn, this can lead to increased rates of stress in the household, divorce, and social isolation. The most insidious aspect of compassion fatigue is that it attacks the very core of what brings helpers into this work: their empathy and compassion for others.
~ Charles Figley

For many, this trauma injury can often come and go. Sometimes you have a bad day, or week, or month. In the heroic fields of public safety, trying to overcome or push away the days where these symptoms come up can quickly lead to unhealthy coping choices, such as excess consumptions; inappropriate actions or negative emotional spiraling that can lead to further health complications like, anxiety/hypervigilance; depression; PTSD; or suicidal thoughts. This is where all our prevention and mitigation tactics like mindfulness, emotional intelligence, combating cognitive distortions, and strategic communications can be a powerful ally in preparing for and overcoming the mental ambush of stress injuries.

The long-term effects of compassion fatigue or burnout can severely hinder a person from being able to care for or even empathize with others, leading to safety concerns, higher absenteeism, and apathy towards those we serve.

Have you struggled with maintaining empathy with those you interact with during their worst possible moments?

____

____

____

____

MANAGING COMPASSION FATIGUE:

- Make time for yourself through self-care. Regularly plan for peace, love, and joy.
- Manage your family-work balance. Set work boundaries and don't overcommit. Be aware of what's meaningful for you and your family and be consistent.
- Recognize physical/emotional triggers and develop healthy habits to deal with them.
- Develop your emotional intelligence, mindfulness, and inner vs outer control thinking.
- Surround yourself with a support network of mentors, positive peers, and friends.
- Seek resources for counseling and/or training that aim to improve your wellness.
- Distance yourself from negative and emotional inputs around you; including chat groups, media feeds you follow on social media, and entertainment options.
- ***Going Beyond the Call* @GBTC911** only posts positive and helpful material, be part of the change. Post and promote your 'good job' or 'save of the day/week' on our feed.

LEADERSHIP: Organizations should have a media specialist posting daily wins on social media to create a balance in public perception. Only hearing the negatives from command or online can also have a serious job satisfaction or even toxic effect on your people. If you do not have a social media person, then you can ask for volunteers on each shift to post regular positive "shout out-to" updates for the public.

Posting parameters for risk mitigation are commonplace in many organizations and can be adapted to ensure an acceptable framework for posts. This will be well received by younger generations while all will enjoy a good story or pat on the back.

What other options can you think of to balance the good and bad of your job?

____

____

____

____

Create a '***wins and strengths'*** journal to mentally download the good you do. This helps the brain balance the positive and negative impacts of your work. **Journal the following regularly:**

WINS I SAVED … I HELPED … I ASSISTED…	STRENGTHS I HELPED… I SOLVED … I COACHED…

HYPERVIGILANCE

HYPERAROUSAL ON THE WINDOW OF TOLERANCE STRESS SCALE

Vigilance is a good thing; a situational awareness that allows you to be scanning your environment and be instantly ready should someone or something intend harm to yourself, a person or property. In the public safety realm, the feeling that you must be "on" while working makes sense for safety. Mentally fit people have highs and lows, they can turn it down or off, allowing the brain, nervous, and adrenal system to reset. Without proper rest and reset, our body can turn against us. When we are ramped up over extended periods, it becomes harder to shut it off.

Ongoing heightened surveillance and hypersensitivity to everything around you can take a toll on your physical and emotional health. This can turn into an anxiety disorder that can take away from our quality of life. Using coping strategies like mindfulness and cognitive behavior therapy (CBT) can help teach our mind to feel safe while training our brains to stay alert to threats.

List recent times where you were unable to turn down the hypervigilance and enjoy the present moment:

____

____

____

____

How has this impacted your most important relationships?

____

____

____

____

____

Learning to shift that high alert energy into a relaxing, mind and body healing calm will save the slow slide to detached, isolated, and apathetic decline often seen with hypervigilance, anxiety, or PTSD. Regular practice of breathing and grounding exercises throughout your shift will help your body get rid of built-up stress chemicals as they happen. Learn to trust your trained subconscious "people reader." We can program what to be alert for and let it do its job, releasing that cognitive burden from your brain when situational assessments provide "all clear" to do so. Learning mindfulness exercises, meditation and body release tactics can also help "let it go" when the shift ends and settle back into a normal level vigilance.

Hypervigilance shows as:

Difficulty sleeping; waking at night and unable to go back to sleep	Unwillingness to engage in conversations or activities not related to work	Intensely alert to, and focused on any conceivable imminent danger
May have outbursts of extreme rage / verbal aggression	Overly alert and suspicious of everyone	On edge or keyed up. A regular sense of dread
Perpetual sense of dread and of being under threat danger	Paranoia possible when frequently perceiving danger in situations where no such danger exists	Difficulty concentrating and mental fogginess
Self-destructive coping choices	Irritable / angry outbursts	Jumpier and easily startled
Reckless / unsafe behavior	Constant anxiety	Panic attacks

If you have been living with hypervigilance a long time you may wish to try assisted treatments. Cognitive Behavior Techniques (CBT) typically runs for 12-16 sessions and focuses on the connective relationship between thoughts, feelings, and one's behaviors. When we can control unhelpful thinking patterns and make better coping choices, it leads to healthier, more balanced behavior and emotional regulation.

We have several mindfulness and grounding exercises in this workbook including deep breathing; yoga or stretching; tense and release exercises; self-hypnosis; reading; and let's consider a big hypervigilance buster, sleep hygiene. A good sleep is essential to every aspect of our health and shift work makes getting a good rest challenging to begin with. Hypervigilance makes this even more difficult; how do you drift off when you are wired for danger? Your body temperature naturally decreases to initiate sleep so keep your sleep space between 60-67-degrees Fahrenheit to promote sleep. The follow habits will also help with resting well off-shift:

- No blue light screens, flashing of games as they stimulate your subconscious. Avoid screens an hour before bed and use *do not disturb* on your phone for your sleep duration. You can always favorite people to ring through if they may need you '*urgently'*.
- Within your shift cycles have a consistent sleep/wake cycle to create a sleeping routine.
- Create night when sleeping during lit hours using blackout curtains, noise dampening devices (white, pink, brown), have rules for non-disturbance, and hide clock.
- Exercise regularly, for some yoga or stretching right before bed works; for many they need a couple hours for the body to calm down.
- Keep your bedspace an intimacy and sleeping sanctuary, no TV's, phones, laptops, etc.
- Avoid eating a larger meal, drinking alcohol, smoking, or caffeine before your sleep time.
- Set a calming routine, a hot shower, relaxing music, read (no blue screen or TV).
- Invest in a good mattress and pillows, good sleep is a critical hypervigilance buster.

What have you tried to calm your hypervigilance in the past? Has one method worked better than others?

POSITIVE PSYCHOLOGY - LEARNED OPTIMISIM

CHANGING DARK AND DREARY THOUGHTS TO OPTIMISTIC AND REALISTIC ONES

Positive Psychology is about training our brain beyond getting "better" and towards creating the best possible version of ourselves to advancing our happiness, peace, and joy experiences. Watch this YouTube describing ***Martin Seligman*** (co-founder of positive psychology and author of "***Training the Brain to Change,"*** youtu.be/1qJvS8v0TTI, also youtu.be/9FBxfd7DL3E. Also,
"*The University of Pennsylvania's* Authentic Happiness" website has a series of happiness satisfaction quizzes: https://www.authentichappiness.sas.upenn.edu/testcenter

When negative spiraling occurs, use this work sheet to journal an upward positive perspective, lesson learned, or a stress releasing version of events:

ADVERSE EVENT	
ADVERSITY FEELING?	
EXPLANITORY BELIEF?	
CONSEQUENCES?	
CHALLENGE THOUGHTS: 1. EVIDENCE? 2. ALTERNATIVES? 3. IMPLICATIONS? 4. USEFULNESS?	
LIST NEW WAYS OF EXPLANING	

Get strategic with yourself. We often move through life without any commitment to goals, aspirations, or intentional effort to build healthy, helpful habits. When we lack aim and focused attention, we can often miss the target, muddling through life wondering why we are dissatisfied.

Journal the following chart using this list and other options from the 'strong roots' work:

TARGETED AREA	ALREADY DO WELL	WOULD LIKE TO DEVELOP	WOULD LIKE TO TRY
Professional			
Relationships			
Emotional			
Spiritual			
Physical			

ACUTE STRESS DISORDER (ASD)
A NORMAL RESPONSE TO AN ABNORMAL SITUATION

Some of you reading this feel they are highly resilient and have all the stress safely locked in a "vault." It is true that many are so resilient that if feels like everything will be fine and it may well be for you. However, for some, that *'one thing'* event happens, and it hits the brain and nervous system hard. This is when preparing for the mental ambush is so very important.

Even if you have managed the same scenario a dozen times, it is critical to recognize that the cumulative stress and trauma can add up and unlock that tightly locked vault. Self-care can do a lot for preventing, mitigating, and managing the stress; and then there are times when we need to acknowledge that professional help is the best option. We are now moving into the arena where the brain and nervous system might require a professional hand to properly reset and get quality of life back on track. You 'may' be able to resolve on your own over time, but life is short; why extend and likely worsen the injury?

Acute Stress Disorder (ASD) is usually notable within 1-3 days and lasts beyond 3 months after a severe stressor. It often involves a feeling of intense fear, hopelessness, or helplessness. It may occur as a direct or indirect/secondary/vicarious trauma and may build from repeated exposure to a reoccurring trauma with a tipping point event. Sufferers may have a hard time recalling specific details of the traumatic event that initiated the ASD response. A person will have notable distress or impairment in social, occupational, or other important interactive and internal areas of functioning.

The American Psychiatric Association's Diagnostic and Statistical Manual of Mental Disorders, Fifth Edition (DSM-5) specifies that, for a diagnosis of ASD, at least nine of 14 symptoms from any of five categories—intrusion, negative mood, dissociation, avoidance, and arousal—must have begun or worsened after the traumatic event. This psychological injury may resolve itself with self-healing, supports, therapy, resilience during this 12-week window. When left untreated, this typically evolves into a more severe disorder, notably, PTSD.

This window of opportunity to avoid a more serious and lasting psychological trauma injury is important for self-care as well as for peers and leadership.

ASD shows as:

A marked decrease in emotional connectivity and responsiveness	Unable to find joy or pleasure in activities, even those previously pursued with vigor	Frequent feelings of guilt even with mundane things
Difficulty concentrating	Numb feeling	World as unreal or dreamlike
Dissociative amnesia	Brain fog/feeling dazed	Depersonalization
Jittery / Fearful	Exaggerated startle response	Difficulty sleeping
Feeling of being detached from body	Avoidance of people, places, conversations	Excessive irritability
Avoiding trauma-related thoughts, emotions	Hypervigilance	Helplessness / Hopelessness

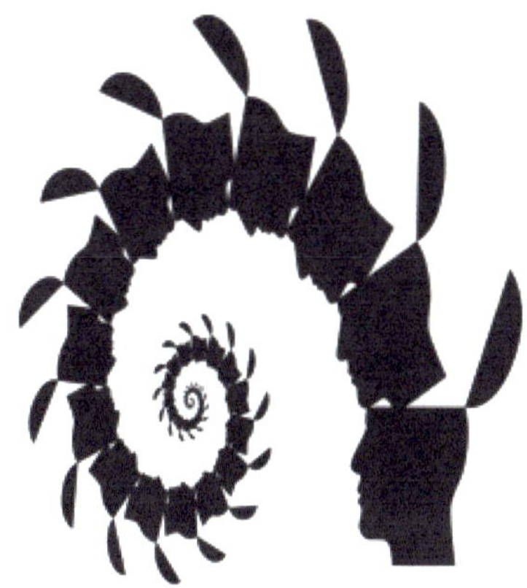

When should you consider seeking help? Although serious and worrisome the physical, interpersonal, cognitive, and emotional reactions (such as grief, guilt, and anger) are normal reactions to abnormal events. One or more of the self-care options, peer-to-peer efforts, critical incident debriefings and other social/relationships connections will often dissipate the heightened stress response. This will depend on your personal resiliency, emotional intelligence, and mental fitness efforts. However, more significant symptoms should raise the alarm that a psychiatric consultation is required to re-set the mental wellness hit received.

These include:

- Dissociative, derealization, fugue, amnesia, and depersonalization symptoms
- Reoccurrence or worsening of addictive or pre-existing mental health issues, or clear
    - substance abuse
- Persistent changes in behavior that is notable and mentioned by loved ones and peers, including, a lack of self-care, hyperarousal, depressive state, or extreme numbness
- Aggressive, violent, or homicidal behavior, or high-risk sexual baiting or aggression
- Intrusive re-experiencing of event(s) including, startling or terrifying memories,
    - flashbacks, and persistent nightmares
- Suicidal thoughts or behaviors that include suicide planning

Have you experienced, or you have seen these heightened reactions in a peer? What did you do about it?

____

____

____

Stress is not always going to be trauma or even job related. Life can be stressful, especially in these times of pandemic outbreaks, political divide, mass shootings, and extreme weather events, to name a few. Score your life stress using the popular Holmes-Rahe Stress Inventory to ensure your wellness goal considers all the influences that may lead to negative mental wellness. https://www.stress.org/holmes-rahe-stress-inventory. Your final score can predict mental and physical health challenges based on common stressors that are piling onto any work-related stress you are bearing.

My Holmes-Rahe Stress Inventory Score was: __________________________

What Does Your Score Mean?

- ***150 points or less: a relatively low amount of life change and a low susceptibility to stress-induced health breakdown***
- ***150 to 300 points: 50% chance of health breakdown in the next 2 years***
- ***300 points or more: 80% chance of health breakdown in the next 2 years, according to the Holmes-Rahe statistical prediction model***

DEPRESSION

Here are five facts about depression everyone needs to know:

1. Depression is not a life sentence.
2. Depression is not a sign of weakness.
3. Depression is not something you "just get over."
4. Depression is not something you should be ashamed of.
5. If you suffer from depression, you are not a failure, weak or defective.

Depression shows as:

These feelings wreak havoc on the mind, body, and soul. Depression sneaks in slowly, a chemical deficiency that shows with minor mood changes, then getting progressively worse, until one day in a worst-case scenario the person wonders, what is the use in living?

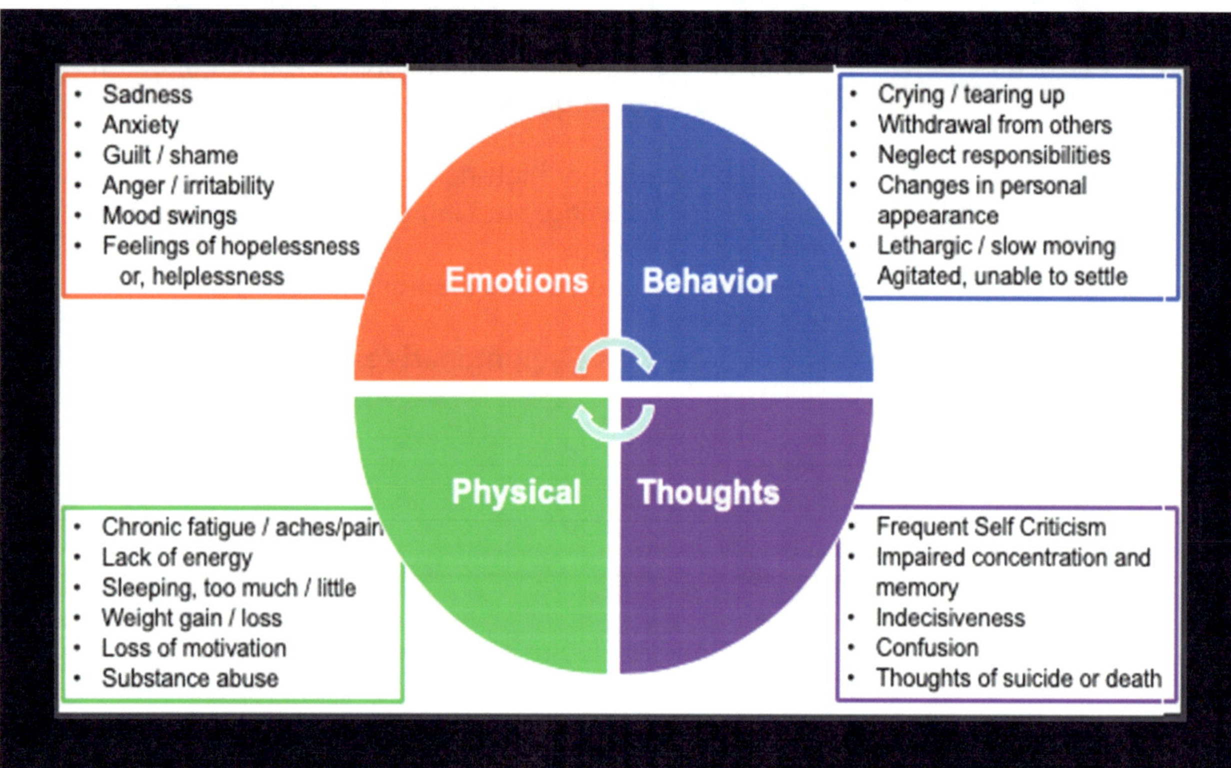

We learned that traumatic stress has a specific effect on our nervous system responsiveness that leads to health problems. Depression has a similar startling impact on brain health. Not only from a psychological perspective, but the ability to affect physical structures in the brain from inflammation and oxygen restriction to actual shrinking. The longer it is left untreated, the more the negative impact and the longer repair and chemical balance needs to reset.

Researchers have proven that the amygdala, thalamus, hippocampus, frontal, and the prefrontal cortex can be affected. The amount of damage is linked to how long the depression has set in and the severity of it, with notable differences showing around 8-12 months. When these areas of our brain shrink, then the optimized functioning also dissipates. Depression changes a person's emotional responses, their ability to recognize social and emotional cues in other people and reduces empathy or other focus. Damage to the hippocampus reduces the functionality of memory processing, which could lead to PTSD with repeated triggers or traumatic incidents.

When you are suffering from depression, all this may be hard to self-evaluate. It tends to sneak in with lowering serotonin chemicals. People go from feeling crappy to feeling like a failure, or hopelessness which may spiral down to suicidal tendencies. Chronic depression can make one feel like a burden to those who care about them and believe they no longer have value to offer.

DEPRESSION QUIZ *Instructions: Answer the questions on how you have behaved and felt* ***during the past week****.*	0 Not at all	1 Just a little	2 Some -what	3 Moderate	4 Quite a lot	5 Very much
I do things slowly.						
My future seems hopeless.						
It is hard for me to concentrate on reading.						
The pleasure and joy, has gone out of my life.						
I have difficulty making decisions.						
I have lost interest in aspects of life that used to be important to me.						
I feel sad, blue, and unhappy.						
I am agitated and keep moving around.						
I feel fatigued.						
It takes great effort for me to do simple things.						
I feel that I am a guilty person who deserves to be punished.						
I feel like a failure.						
I feel lifeless -- more dead than alive.						
My sleep has been disturbed, too little, too much, or broken sleep.						
I spend time thinking about HOW I might kill myself.						
I feel trapped or caught.						
I feel depressed even when good things happen to me.						
Without trying to diet, I have lost, or gained, weight.						
TOTALS						
SCORE						

Score	Result	Score	Result
0-9	No depression likely	22-35	Mild to moderate depression
10-17.	Possible mild depression	36-53.	Moderate to severe depression
18-21.	Borderline depression	54-up.	Severe depression

What supports have I investigated and have at the ready for myself, a peer or a loved one to get the help needed when depression is indicated? Add to the chart.

People Supports	Lifestyle	Spiritual	Emotional / Mental	Physical
Family	Structure/Routine	Prayer	Positive self-talk	Nutrition
Friends	Relaxation	Meditation	Positive cognitive work	Proper sleep
Psychiatrist	Fulfilling activity	Spiritual community	Journaling / mood log	Exercise
Therapist	Positive sexual relationship	Forgiveness	Therapist	Water ++++++
Chaplain	Setting goals	Finding purpose	Supportive group/friends	Medication
Support Group	Planned pleasure	Mindfulness	Emotional Intelligence	Supplements
Positive outings with positive people	Spending time in nature	Giving back to community	Effective Communication skills	Breathing and Grounding exercises

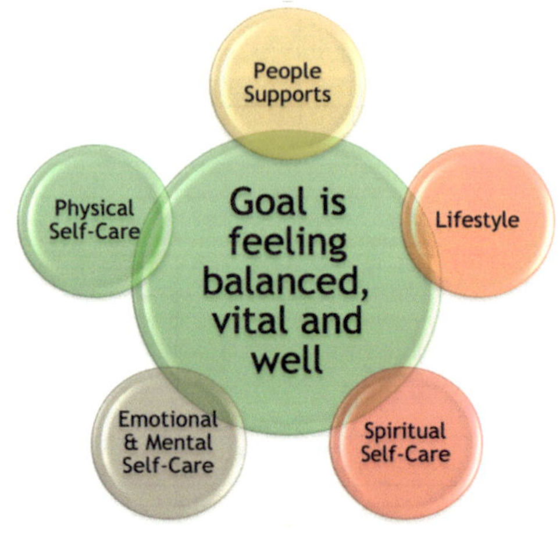

What areas do I commit to prioritizing to expand and grow?

1. ______________________________

2. ______________________________

3. ______________________________

4. ______________________________

5. ______________________________

Is there an area I believe having an accountability partner will help me to achieve my new wellness roots? Who will I ask to help me succeed?

____

____

POST TRAUMATIC STRESS DISORDER (PTSD)
(Chapter 2 and 8)

"PTSD may be one of the most preventable of psychiatric disorders. There are interventions effective in preventing PTSD shortly after a person experiences a traumatic event. They are too resource-intensive to give to everyone." Laramie Duncan, ~Stanford University.

PTSD is not a new mental health issue, first brought to public attention in psychological history as shell shock in WWI, it has a disturbing initiation as a mass political cover up. Our book provides a longer version in Chapter 2 – Stigma Busting. The governing body and a medical expert conspired to make 'shell shock' a lack of manliness issue versus a medical condition because they could not afford the pension and health care needs of returning soldiers. By such labeling they could deny pensions and embarrass soldiers into avoiding discussion about the effects of war. This traumatic stress injury has gone through a few name changes in following conflicts, settling on PTSD after the Vietnam War. After returning soldiers joined first responder roles across the nation, they brought the 'stigma' of acute stress and PTSD being a weakness versus a psychological wound that needed treatment to heal.

An official diagnosis did not form until 1980 when it was included in the Diagnostic and Statistical Manual of Mental Disorders, 3rd edition (DSM-III), descriptions of clusters of symptoms in response to trauma have been noted for many years. It is not limited to soldiers – PTSD symptoms can develop in individuals from all walks of life exposed to different types of traumas (some examples include motor vehicle accident, assault, natural disaster).

Does this history alter the way you have perceived PTSD?

____

____

So, what exactly is PTSD? As per the DSM-5, symptoms can be grouped into clusters, which include:

- Intrusive – these might include memories, nightmares, triggers
- Avoidance of memories or triggers
- Negative changes in thoughts or mood – these might include negative beliefs about self or others, blaming of self or others, forgetting parts of the trauma, persistent negative emotions, emotional numbing, detachment from others, loss of interest in things normally enjoyed
- Marked changes in arousal and reactivity – these might include irritability, recklessness, hypervigilance, strong startle response, concentration, or sleep difficulties

What constitutes a psychological "trauma" can vary somewhat, but it typically involves witnessing deaths of others, or experiencing or witnessing violence or significant threats to the safety of oneself or another. The very nature of first responders' work lends itself to exposure to potentially traumatic incidents on a regular basis.

How many times have you experienced or witnessed events that could have created a psychological injury during your career (including past experiences in the military or childhood)?

___

___

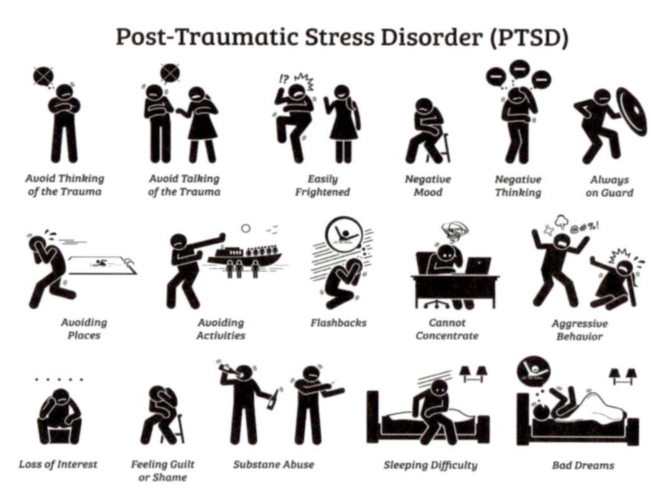

IMAGE FROM: heroesmile.com

Public safety careers take a toll on your soul, yet our amazing selfless public servants are not well prepared for the mental ambush. In more recent years the military has done a better job at preparing their warriors for the events, experiences, and effects of battle. They have improved their post event support options as well, knowing no one walks away from in-theatre warfare without a few soul-searing scars. So, let's work together to bust the stigma and build stronger internal response systems to this known enemy.

Whether you are in one of the responder roles, emergency medical, forensic, and other investigative or military positions. Post incident roles within justice, disaster, mass causality, and search and rescue. To the longer-term impact from positions in victim support, specialty investigative units, child services, and corrections who manage the worst of humanity as they interact in a high threat, primal environment that keeps them highly vigilant for theirs and others safety. All will feel the mental ambush at one time or many times throughout their career.

We can all understand the impact of direct trauma when it happens TO you. It is the other types that stealthily attack unseen until it's too late. You are not only managing the impact of someone else's horrific moment; your brain and nervous systems are being invaded with bits and pieces of soul sucking input merely by proximity. This work, by definition, often involves primary or tertiary witness to deaths, horrors, and injuries.

The number of potentially traumatic scenes exposed to in one shift may be more than what most people would experience in their lifetime. While they may become used to such scenes, particular calls may cause more distress, such as the deaths or major injuries of children, coming across someone who looks like someone they love, or a particularly nasty reminder of human depravity or stupidity.

These professionals typically work in a "suck it up" culture – not only for others, but for themselves as well. Thus, various types of stress reactions or even posttraumatic symptoms can gradually and progressively build up over time. Increasing numbers of traumatic incidents can result in *cumulative trauma*. The stigma associated with being a "rescuer" who then asks for help has tended to be prevalent in first responder organizations and can be a significant barrier to seeking much needed help.

Have you ever felt overwhelmed with what you have witnessed or managed at a scene and felt you had to swallow it down and ignore your very human reaction to unthinkable sensory inputs?

____

____

Other factors can impact emotional reactivity and distress as well. Consider shift work, extreme fatigue, disruptions to family and social lives, and lacking availability or acceptance in organizational support. Factor in a common deep mistrust of the confidentiality of getting help and the career impacting aspects of word getting out and help becomes a four-letter word. Often, first responders may continue to work for a long time despite reduced ability to cope and continue to be routinely exposed to traumatic events.

Eventually, they may reach a "breaking point," that "one thing" that cracks the emotional vault, even after what may appear to be a relatively minor event. A comparison can be made to injuring one's ankle. If one continues to walk on the ankle without allowing it to heal, the ankle may become vulnerable to re-injury, even to lighter levels of stress. Without proper care the ability to repair the injury to pre-existing strength becomes harder and longer with continued neglect.

Historically, first responders have, at times, had trouble having this cumulative impact of stress recognized by employers and worker's compensation boards. Some have had compensation claims denied due to difficulty identifying one single event that could be considered atypical or considerable in a first responder's work duties that contributed to the PTSD. One practical reason why documenting, seeking help or council, even sharing with a trusted advisor within your organization can help when the build-up becomes unmanageable.

Does this understanding change how you have perceived PTSD in the past? Does it ring true for you or someone you work with? How will you interpret this disorder differently now?

____

____

____

DEEPER DIVE ON PTSD

One time or cumulative traumatic injury responses are processed through the limbic system (emotional control center) and stored in the hippocampus (brain library) where they are converted into long term memory. When one or more of these experiences has a heightened emotional element, it may linger or what we often call "spin" in our minds and fail to process properly to long term memory. This is true of all ultra-heightened emotional responses. Whether it is the blind euphoria of new love, an amazing and personally impacting experience, or the horror of a traumatic event. When it processes correctly and moves into long term memory you can still recall the event, or see, smell, taste, hear things that trigger it, but it does not necessarily take over thinking.

For traumatic stress injuries that lead to PTSD, there is a 4-12-week window where resilience, awareness, prevention, mitigation, and calming techniques can help provide psychological first aid to move memories into long term memory.

PTSD on the other hand, once set in, often includes a looped playback, a tunnel vision perspective of an aspect of the memory that particularly triggered you. It is not processed properly so it manifests as a live recurrence and all those triggers are felt as if it just happened, not as a memory.

While PTSD may be caused by one specific event, ***Dr. Hartman*** created this chart that expresses a typical cumulative aspect of PTSD.

We strongly recommend seeking help if you feel you are on the PTSD cumulative ladder. Have a professional help you RESET your brain works fast to get you back on track to be able to self-manage your mental fitness well.

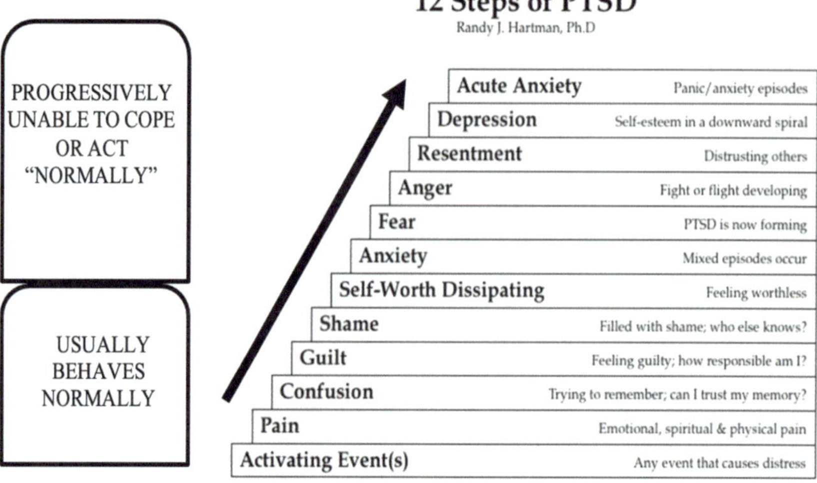

One way to help peers through a traumatic event is communicate as soon as possible i.e., "wow that scene was messed up, how are you doing with it?" If they happen to describe one element of a particularly disturbing memory, then interrupt them with questions that expand that memory, expand from a microfocus to a broader perspective. Ask about the color of the walls, weather outside, was there a car in the driveway or not? Ask who was beside them, were they on the left or right … basically any odd or irrelevant questions that require they pull themselves out of their hyper-focused thought and think about the answer. Asking these types of questions bumps them from their emotional limbic center to their cognitive (rational) brain to respond, interrupting the spinning that can cause so much damage to the psyche. It's okay that they know why you are doing this, say "hey, that's a really painful focus you have going on, I'm going to ask you some questions to broaden that hyper-focused memory."

Have you seen yourself or a peer on this tiered ladder before? How did you manage? Who did you reach out to? Have you reached out at all or are you still battling the demons? Will you change how you manage this now? How will you manage peers when they show signs of psychological trauma?

____

____

____

Post-Traumatic Stress Disorder (PTSD) shows as:

RE-EXPERIENCING	AVOIDANCE	HYPER/HYPO AROUSAL
Unwelcome memories	Emotional numbing	Agitated over small things
Replaying and beating up self over choices, decisions	Reduced awareness of one's surroundings	Trouble getting or staying asleep
Nightmares	Depersonalization	Jittery/ Easily startled
Spontaneous memories	Sense of suffering	Increased wariness/distrust
Flashbacks	Overwhelming guilt or shame	On-alert for danger
Triggers from any reminders	Disconnected or detached	Hyperactivity
What-if scenarios	Amnesia / loss of memory	Always on edge
Self or others due to a distorted sense of reality	Avoid people that give you association to event	Extreme sensitivity to light and sounds
Blaming	Burying distressing thoughts	Moodiness or mood swings
Anger towards peers / or others involved	I'm OK response when you're not	May strive to be super busy to avoid thinking
Spiritual anger	Burying feelings	Self-destructive behavior
Anger towards the organization, establishment, system etc.	Avoiding external reminders of the event	Increased sexual energy, risky behavior
Negative thoughts about yourself, other people, or the world	Feeling isolated & alone	Recklessness
Event takes predominance in mind over relationships	Disconnection from others including family/trusted friends	Anxiety/Panic/Phobias
Self and other critical	Uninterested in usual hobbies	Depression
Difficulty experiencing positive emotions	Sexual disinterest / Erectile issues	Depressive episodes
Difficulty maintaining close relationships	Trouble concentrating	Fears & helplessness

Within these professions you are apt to feel any one or a few of these emotions at various times while managing the stress of the job. Know you need help when it starts to impact your quality of life, relationships, and personal health.

____

____

____

____

COMPLEX PTSD (C-PTSD)

C-PTSD falls under Disorders of Extreme Stress Not Otherwise Specified (DESNOS) and is commonly associated to extreme childhood abuse, repeated sexual assault, or abandonment. It is also a diagnosis potential for those who suffer from chronic trauma repeated over months or years, including POWs, or public safety professionals who are repeatedly exposed to the worst of humanity and traumatic experiences.

Generally, C-PTSD is only diagnosed after treatment has started for something else, and specific behavioral indices are noted. It shows most often with a borderline or antisocial personality disorder or dissociative disorders. C-PTSD diagnosis commonly shows a severe negative self-image and an inability to affect regulation (unable to cope with extreme emotions like anger or sadness), severe emotional distrust and for some a loss of faith in humanity. C-PTSD sufferers may also experience a preoccupation with revenge against their abuser or for some, obsession with the criminal element responsible for a tragic situation. Given most of the symptom's mirror those of PTSD, victims are often misdiagnosed, and treatments are ineffective. This may manifest in self-blame for the sufferer/victim or futility that nothing can help them instead of knowledge that the diagnosis and treatment may be wrong.

Have you or someone you know been diagnosed with PTSD and found treatment ineffective? Do you feel a professional with C-PTSD experience might be a better option?

____

____

____

If you are partnered with someone with C-PTSD, their emotions can be unpredictable, extreme and flare up without reason. This seemingly disproportional emotional responsiveness often has root in extreme childhood neglect or abuse on top of current cumulative traumatic impacts. It may leave that sufferer/victim feeling worthless, unlovable, helpless, and empty. This void and often accompanying hunger, anxiety, and fear takes precedence over other logic or feelings.

Outbursts are commonly followed with an intense need to self-medicate with the chosen self-harming option they use. You will run into increased cases of C-PTSD victims while working in underprivileged communities where often generational trauma perpetuates child abuse and sexual assault. Also with sex trade workers, sex slave victims and rape victims with a background of abuse.

Additionally, a person with this disorder commonly has difficulties in forming and maintaining healthy relationships. Sexual abuse may show in risky and self-destructing behaviors, and often eating disorders, which are also common to rape victims. Self-harming or extreme risk behaviors create a sense of relief from mental anguish, similar to those whose addictions are drugs or alcohol. C-PTSD may show as a series of self-harming behaviors or a lifestyle of risky choices that act as self- medication like sexual addiction, gambling, eating disorders, self-harm, cutting, and various substance abuse.

COMPLEX POST TRAUMATIC STRESS DISORDER (C-PTSD) shows as:

Severe negative self-image	Feeling unlovable, worthless	Avoidance behaviors
Trouble forming and keeping relationships	Depersonalization	Loss of one's core beliefs, values, religious faith
Alcohol or drug abuse	Sexual acting out	Aggression
Impulsivity/Outbursts	Eating Disorders	Fragmented thinking
Self-destructive actions	Exaggerated emotional responses (Panic, rage, or depression)	Dissociation and amnesia

Consider some of the community members you have interacted with, or a partner where you just couldn't understand their self-destructive actions. Perhaps this insight is helpful with your own self-care journey? Write down a few examples. Does this knowledge aid your awareness and empathy towards this trauma outcome?

____

____

____

____

____

____

Once PTSD sets in the most beneficial action for someone to take is getting professional help to re-set their emotional, chemical, and nervous system responses. Self-care strategies in conjunction with professional support may also be beneficial.

Public safety professionals can take recommendations for self-care from leading organizations like the National Center for PTSD/C-PTSD. We have chosen a few and expanded on them:

- Regularly check-in with colleagues, family, and friends. Having a circle of trust and confidence helps work through issues that build due to emotional and negative thinking.
- Utilize a group if you would prefer privacy, there are many online specific to first responders.
- Help partners or teams understand the PTSD/C-PTSD diagnosis. Helping them keep an eye out and avoid aggravating any triggers will allow them to support an improved outcome.
- Practice relaxation techniques and stress management breaks. If you are in a leadership role, make this practice part of shift briefings to remove any stigma associated to good mental health.
- Periodically check in with a peer, Chaplain, mental health support and a trusted leadership link for consultation. Work together to manage crisis incidents.

- Learn to manage anxieties towards actual threats – mindfulness, journaling and working on multiple interpretations to any perceived worry can help narrow down the good-bad-ugly outlook and lessen extreme or runaway thinking.
- Work to maintain helpful self-talk – challenge yourself the way you would challenge loved ones, partners, or friends if they were beating themselves up.
- Focus effort on what is within one's power and control to fix, change or influence.
- Foster a spirit of endurance, patience, tolerance, and hope.

While doing all the above public safety professionals should avoid the following:

- Working too long by themselves without checking in with colleagues
- Working "round the clock" with few breaks
- Feeling that they are not doing enough
- Excessive intake of sweets, nicotine, and caffeine
- Engaging in self-talk and attitudinal obstacles to self-care

What other self-care options have you heard about, tried or are curious about?

____

____

____

Testing and Treatment Supports USA:

PTSD: https://itherapy.com/interactive-ptsd-self-assessment/ (Also has a "find a therapist" link)

U.S. Department of Veteran Affairs site National Center for PTSD for self-tests, knowledge links, and support groups. https://www.ptsd.va.gov/index.asp

PTSD Treatment Decision Aid (https://www.ptsd.va.gov/apps/decisionaid/) helps to understand more about different therapies

TREATMENT LOCATOR: https://findtreatment.samhsa

The Birdwell Foundation supports our work and has great programs at https://www.birdwellfoundation.org/blog/911-first-responders-get-help-with-birdwell-foundation

Look up local PTSD/C-PTSD support options and list them here for future reference:

____

____

____

____

PTSD TREATMENT OPTIONS

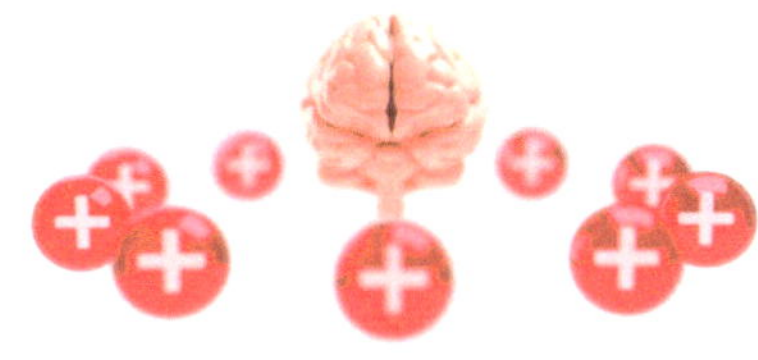

There are many treatment options available pending your personal interest and comfort in non- medical or alternative options.

Psychotherapy - Cognitive behavioral therapy (CBT) is a style of talk-therapy that focuses on the relationship between thoughts, feelings, and behaviors. CBT targets current symptoms and problems, usually lasting 12-16 sessions and can be done in an individual or group format.

Cognitive Processing Therapy – A specific CBT therapy that focuses on how your traumatic event is perceived and your self-driven coping choices to manage the emotional and mental part of your experience.

EMDR – Eye movement desensitization and reprocessing techniques utilizes bilateral sensory input such as side-to-side eye movements to help you process difficult memories, thoughts, and emotions related to your trauma.

Hypnotherapy - or clinical hypnosis, is a solution-oriented therapy treatment that works with a person's conscious and subconscious minds to elicit emotional and behavioral change. It has been found to be effective when treating such issues as anxiety, stress, phobias, and post-traumatic stress disorder (PTSD). It seems most effective when combined with CBT.

Acupuncture – An eastern medicine energy practice that involves inserting thin needles into certain areas of the body to help prevent or relieve health issues. Approved by the Department of Veterans Affairs as an approved complementary and alternative medicine treatment for PTSD, studies have shown acupuncture to be safe and cost-effective.

Chiropractic / Massage – Tension and misalignment are common to high stress body impacts. Prioritizing your physiological health will help you focus on other psychological wellness aspects.

Virtual Reality Exposure - Exposure therapy (VRET) offers the technology for you to be gradually exposed to your traumatic situation while working closely with a trained clinician.

Medications – Medication for PTSD target the brain's threat-processing systems. The goal is to reduce intrusive symptoms along with any depressive and anxiety symptoms that accompany them. Selective serotonin reuptake inhibitors (SSRIs) and serotonin-norepinephrine reuptake inhibitors (SNRIs) are commonly used to treat both depression and anxiety and have been used effectively for PTSD. They help to lower anxious rumination, improve emotional range, reduce intrusive symptoms, and help one feel less irritable and on edge.

***Fluoxetine (Prozac).** Prozac can effectively alleviate symptoms of depression within a week and is a safe and effective medication for a wide range of people. Prozac for PTSD is a good choice for people with serious cognitive symptoms who want to improve their mental clarity and emotional responsiveness. It is a particularly good choice for people with comorbid PTSD and major depressive disorder.

***Paroxetine (Paxil).** Paxil is an SSRI that is used to treat both depression and anxiety. Paxil for PTSD will help people with significant avoidance symptoms and especially for those with comorbid anxiety disorders. Studies have shown that it can effectively address the full range of PTSD symptoms, including intrusive symptoms.

***Sertraline (Zoloft).** Zoloft is the first drug approved by the Food and Drug Administration for the specific treatment of PTSD. It is an effective choice for people looking for a single medication that can treat the full range of PTSD symptoms, including intrusive symptoms. Zoloft is effective for treating numbing and hyperarousal symptoms.

Venlafaxine (Effexor). Effexor effectively addresses avoidance, numbing and re-experiencing symptoms. Research shows that it is helpful for people with comorbid PTSD and depression. It is strongly recommended for the treatment of PTSD by the U.S. Department of Defense and Department of Veterans Affairs (VA).

**It is worth noting that sexual side effects are among the most common complaints about antidepressants for both men and women, the starred ones above having the highest complaints. It is important to communicate with your significant other about this potential and work together on solutions that work for both of you. Raising levels of serotonin in the body allows a feeling of calm and less anxiety which is important to reset your system. It may prevent the hormones that cause our bodies to respond to sex from transmitting their message to our brains and our libido. Medication may dial down one's sex drive, cause delayed or blocked orgasm, lessen ability to lubricate in women or ability to achieve or maintain an erection for men. Some studies indicate a potential increase in birth defects and lower sperm counts as well, so starting or adding to a family is worth discussing with your doctor.*

Stellate Ganglion Block (SGB)

A new procedure that eases symptoms to allow the recipient time to work through underlying issues. The Stellate Ganglion Block (SGB) treatment is a widely used procedure shown to provide relief from symptoms like continual sleep disturbance, surges of anxiety and irritability, hypervigilance, difficulties concentrating and jumpiness.

CBD - Cannabidiol or CBD, shows great potential in the treatment of PTSD symptoms. Studies have shown CBD to have efficacy in alleviating and improving various ailments related to the experience of PTSD, including inflammation, levels of the stress hormone cortisol, anxiety, negative mood, depression, hyperactivity, nightmares, sleep disturbances, body pain, the recurring experience of negative thoughts, and anhedonia or the inability to feel pleasure.

****Even without THC additive some CBD oils have been found to have trace amounts of THC in them so always check with your Human Resources department on how this may impact your agencies annual or random drug testing.*

What other options have you heard of? What would you be willing and unwilling to try or at least learn more about?

____

____

____

The most important part of seeking any support is understanding that, like any health care option, it is not a one size fits all situation. It may be necessary to try a few options before finding the one that best matches your brain chemical, nervous system, and personal comfort style. Medication may be required to assist your brain to reset and be capable of benefiting from other treatment options. Often, we don't see the full scale of the problem ourselves. It is imperative therefore to prepare for the mental ambush by including those closest to you in your self-care plan. That may mean listening to people you trust to spot hidden wounds you are not fully aware of or willing to face in the moment.

If friends, peers, or trusted family tell me I am not the same person and I should seek help, list the mental fitness options you would be willing to try.

1. ____
2. ____
3. ____
4. ____
5. ____

Make an accountability commitment to one of your connections to listen and act when they notice and share concerns about changes to your behavior.

While we can develop a better response system to PTSD and C-PTSD, ideally organizational strategy should work towards prevention and lessening occurrences of PTSD. The cost of this preventative strategy, along with reducing potential liability that comes with stress fueled incidents and safety violations, indicates training like ours is the most logical solution.

From an organizational perspective what measures would you like to see your agency take to reduce psychological stress injuries?

____

____

____

____

____

SUICIDE PREVENTION

People who feel suicidal tend to share feelings of hopelessness, helplessness, and depression. They see suicide as a way out of solving their mental anguish, removing the burden of whom they feel they have become, and to eliminate their overwhelming suffering; and often they speak to those feelings in some manner. Although suicide ideation is not always easy to notice, many verbalize warnings or show signs in the time leading up to their death. Sadly, many of us don't know how to recognize those signs, or fail to take them seriously, thinking someone is just blowing off steam.

Suicidal ideation and warnings of helplessness, hopelessness, or worthlessness are not harmless bids for attention; they are important cries for help that should be taken seriously. Remember, you are not there to act as the therapist, only to be the one who observes and acts when someone's health is in jeopardy. Observe both behavioral and verbal clues.

The red circles specifically indicate primary areas of concern with public safety professionals.

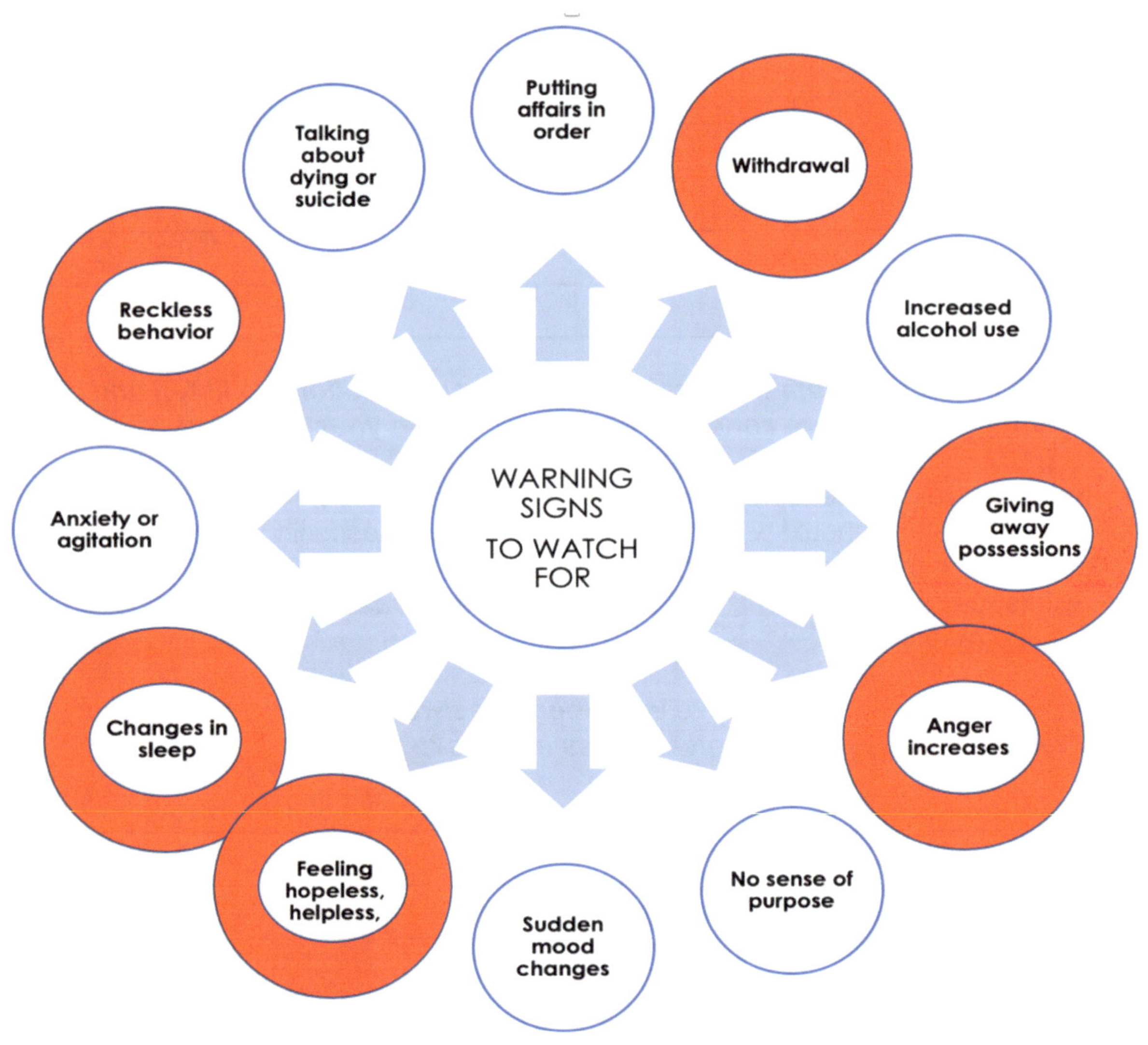

- Verbalizing in conversation or perceived jokes and quips that they feel isolated and lonely.
- Post-retirement chat may talk about a loss of status or importance; having no reason; no purpose; or a sense of loss.
- Depressive comments about a lack of supportive people in one's life, rumination, and negative spinning on problems without solutions.
- Beating themselves up as a failure; generalized expressions of hopelessness, uselessness, notable self- esteem issues.
- Expressing feelings of failure, lack of hope, or loss of self-esteem.
- Talking about a lack of, or loss of, faith, connecting or belief system, like, "things just aren't the same," "God has given up on me," or "I don't fit in anymore." (Change of "Brotherhood or Sisterhood" membership of uniformed service, changes in command, loss of relationships, loss of peers, career changes).
- Whether with a tone of humor or not, discussing a suicide plan, or questioning, "how would you do it?"
- Mentioning a need to or starting to clean up one's affairs and getting things in order.
- Giving away valuable or prized possessions; unusual talk around financial, administrative, wills, burial plots to make it easier for those left behind (again with other signs of depression or traumatic stress).
- A growing removal from social systems, no longer wanting to be around or feeling able to relate to friends, family, peers. Noticeable withdrawal from once enjoyed activities and gatherings.

Have you interacted with someone and based on these warning signs, wondered if they were in crisis?

____

____

____

____

____

____

"But I don't want to be responsible for wrecking someone's career or benching them!" A common reason people tell themselves when they are unsure whether someone is at risk for suicide or just having a bad day, or week. Calling a Chaplain when you are unsure is a great way for them to get anonymous, safe, counselling before more direct action when you are unsure.

If someone has opened the communication door directly or indirectly on the issue of suicide, the Columbia Suicide Severity Rating Scale (C-SSRS) has a few short questions you can ask. This tool helps assess someone and can help you confirm that action is needed to help the person. It has been showing great results with students as well as the military. After putting the C-SSRS in everybody's hands, the U.S. Marine Corps reduced the number of service member suicides by 22%.

Columbia Suicide Severity Rating Scale (C-SSRS)

1. Have you wished you were dead or wished you could go to sleep and not wake up?
2. Have you had any thoughts about killing yourself? If no, go to #6
3. Have you thought about how you might do this?
4. Have you had any intention of acting on these thoughts of killing yourself, as opposed to having the thoughts, but you definitely would not act on them? (HIGH RISK)
5. Have you started to work out or worked out the details of how to kill yourself? Do you intend to carry out this plan? (HIGH RISK)
6. Have you done anything, started to do anything, or prepared to do anything to end your life? (E.g., collected pills, obtained a gun, gave away valuables, wrote a will or suicide note, held a gun to your head but changed your mind, cut yourself, tried to hang yourself, etc.? (HIGH RISK if in last 3 months, medium risk otherwise).

Yes, to any high-risk question indicates the need for further care. Please do not leave the person alone, get family, a counselor, or a close friend on the scene to manage the next steps, or escort them to professional help. Do not believe them if they say they will seek help on their own. Call the national suicide prevention lifeline for options of care **1-800-273-8255 (TALK) or call the new 988 national suicide and crisis lifeline** or check the list of some other support options at the end of the chapter. Suicide may be averted with the right care and treatment. Add these and other hotline numbers into your cell for easy access when you or a peer needs help.

A helpful chart for PEER-to-PEER, leadership, and self-evaluation has been adapted for your use from the Canadian Armed Forces Mental Continuum Model.

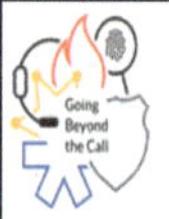

GBTC911.com

Prepare for the Mental Ambush Health Continuum Model

Healthy	Reacting	Injured	Trauma
Regular mood fluctuations	Irritability, sadness, nervousness, moody	Anger, Anxiety, hopelessness, pervasive sadness	Excessive anxiety, quick to anger, rage, consistent depressed mood
Healthy sleep patterns	Tired, low energy, muscle tension, headaches / illness	Disturbed or restless sleep	Difficulty falling or staying asleep, never feeling rested
Consistent performance	Procrastination, avoidance	Non-present in work, social activities, performance lacking	Unable to perform to standards, disciplinary actions, increased absence
Socially active	Decreasing social and hobby activity	Social withdrawal, people avoidance	Isolation, avoiding social events and people once enjoyed
Physically active, healthy mindset	Skipping workouts, active pursuits	Avoiding exercise, active pursuits, very low energy	Exhaustion, regular physical illnesses, injuries
ACTIONS TO TAKE AT EACH PHASE OF THE CONTINUUM			
Prepare for the mental ambush with education	Recognize limits, build in self-care	Seek help and act on your root system plan, journal stressors	Seek professional brain health supports, doctor and counselling
Break down problems into manageable chunks	Plan better rest, exercise and food intake	Reach out to best choice on your SOS call list to talk it out	Utilize recommended counselling actions to get back on track
Grow emotional intelligence and support systems, build your top 3 call list	Utilize mindfulness, and healthy coping strategies	Break up duties and tasks into smaller chunks/actions, prioritize, defer, delete lesser tasks	Seek family/friend support to build in healthier lifestyle options,
Maintain a healthy root system	Identify stressors and implement actions to minimize or counter them	Commit to regular social interactions even when you don't want to	Plan consistent social interplay (even group support initially)

ADDICTION - SUBSTANCE AND BEHAVIOR

WATCH: "The opposite of addiction isn't sobriety. It's connection." Johann Hari, TEDTALK Everything you know about addiction is wrong

"A hurt is at the center of all addictive behaviors. It is present in the gambler, the internet addict, the compulsive shopper, and the workaholic." Gabor Mat, author: "In the Realm of the Hungry Ghosts: Close Encounters with Addiction."

An addictive disorder is an illness that can affect anyone. No definitive answer explains why some become addicted while others do not, but genetics has been proven to play a role. There are many studies also linking psychological disorders, stress, and environmental contributors show increased addictive outcomes. Addiction is a brain disorder associated with physical changes to your brain circuits that involve reward and pleasure seeking, learning, decision-making, self-control, and stress activity. Substances and addictive behaviors have many different effects on the brain, all produce an increased surge of the pleasure neurotransmitter dopamine. The basal ganglia, the control center for rewards and learning about rewards transmit messages between your nerve cells.

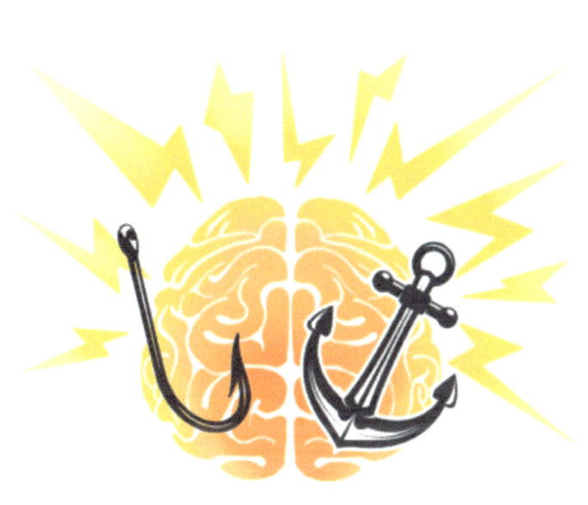

Addiction will progress as neurotransmitters adapt and scale back overwhelming dopamine hits obtained from addictive substances and behaviors and tolerance is built. As the brain alters to maintain balance with the increased presence of dopamine, the user feels an increased hook to chase the desired pleasure response. This is true for drugs, alcohol, gambling, sex, food, high-risk behaviors, shopping, electronics, and other addictive options. The need for more substance or behavior to get the same dopamine hit also means a person will feel less enjoyment in lesser activities that once brought pleasure. The brain's reward center drives a need for the heightened dopamine fix and entices the person to avoid less enjoyable activities and people who do not aid pursuit of the addictive activity.

Willpower is often not successful as the brain is now acting against our better judgement and control. The amygdala (emotional center) and prefrontal cortex (decision center) are part of our stress response system, but neurotransmitters seeking that dopamine burst from addictive pursuits take over as the priority and push the pursuit of the addictive hook, whatever that is for you.

Researchers have found that addiction over a long period begins to change the brain in critical and lasting ways. This point is different for everyone, but it is like a switch is turned on and you cross the line from heavy use to dependence on the addictive hook that starts to become an anchor. Your addiction or behavior begins to take priority over other areas of your life and relationships, employment, and quality of life take a back seat to that substance or behavior that compels you, regardless of the cost to the rest of your life.

SAMHSA's National Helpline, 1-800-662-HELP (4357) (also known as the Treatment Referral Routing Service), or TTY: 1-800-487-4889 is a confidential, free, 24-hour-a-day, 365-day-a-year, information service. This service provides referrals to local treatment facilities, support groups, and community-based organizations.

Also visit the online treatment locator, or send your zip code via text message: 435748 (HELP4U) to find help near you. Read more about the HELP4U text messaging service.

How do you manage event after event; observing what addiction does to other people's lives and wellbeing then go home, look in the mirror, and recognize the same slippery slope in our own reflection? Or with a close or respected peer?

____

____

____

____

Determining when substance *use* morphs to abuse, then addiction, can be challenging and best discussed with a medical professional. For substance use disorders (SUD) they will turn to the Diagnostic and Statistical Manual of Mental Disorders, 5th Edition (DSM-5). The following questions are adapted from the DSM-5 criteria to help you determine whether you should seek help overcoming a substance or behavioral activity that does not serve your wellness goals.

SUBSTANCE ABUSE QUIZ (drugs refer to prescription and non-prescription)	**YES**	**NO**
Do you regularly use alcohol or drugs for something other than a medical reason?		
When you use alcohol or drugs, do you regularly mix to get a better buzz?		
Have you ever felt that you ought to cut down on your drinking or drug use?		
Have people annoyed you by repeatedly criticizing your drinking or drug use?		
Do you find yourself preoccupied with when you can next drink or use drugs?		
Is your home life negatively impacted because of your alcohol or drug use?		
Are you in jeopardy of losing your friends, significant other, family due to use?		
Do you need to drink or use drugs to have fun or to enhance your social life?		
Has your job performance or status been negatively impacted by use?		
Do you lie about or hide the amount you drink or use?		
Do you regularly drink or use drugs while you are alone?		
Have you had repeated loss of memory due to drinking or drug use?		
Do you use drugs or drink to cope with trauma pain, anger, anxiety, or depression?		
Do you regularly take medication beyond the dosage prescribed?		
Have you gone to multiple physicians to get the same medications?		
Do you regularly feel bad or guilty about your drinking or drug use?		
Is your home life unhappy because of your drug or alcohol use?		
Do you drink or use drugs upon waking to steady your nerves or to get rid of a hangover?		
Yes, to any one of these is a sign to consider talking to a professional		

Substance Abuse Rates Among Firefighters

Drug Abuse Rates

10%

Alcohol Abuse Rates

29%

Two in Five EMTs engage in high-risk use drugs and alcohol

Police Officer Alcoholism Rates

After Two Years on the Force

27%

After Four Years on the Force

36%

At the time of writing there were not any definitive statistics on Communications, Corrections, or Forensics to show. However, we can estimate a higher-than-average consumption based on other statistics found for depression, anxiety, and suicidal tendencies. (https://sbtreatment.com/resources/first-responders-guide/)

As a peer, or leader, in these high stress organizations, some of these quiz questions can become part of your behavioral mindfulness when observing or looking out for a member under your care. For performance evaluations, these questions can also raise awareness of when mandatory counselling may be an effective option before career-limiting actions place a member's life in a dire situation or impact the safety of other team members.

Does this test make you rethink whether a perceived habit or coping mechanism has moved into a danger zone for you?

____

____

____

____

If yes, what action(s) will you commit to manage a healthier you?

____

____

____

____

Is there a peer or member under your charge that comes to mind when reviewing these questions?

____

____

____

____

____

BEYOND COMMON SUBSTANCE DISORDERS

Behavior addictions are also common with high stress professions. Here are links to help you self-assess and determine the best course of action for accepting and addressing behaviors that are not helping your mental fitness and wellness goals. ***PSYCHOLOGY TOOLS .com*** has many tests you can utilize for a reality check on when a coping habit is moving towards a danger zone, and you need to pay attention. Here are few:

GAMBLING: https://psychology-tools.com/test/nods-clip

GAMING: https://psychology-tools.com/test/excessive-gaming-screening-tool

SHOPPING: https://psychology-tools.com/test/bergen-shopping-addiction-scale

AGGRESSION: https://psychology-tools.com/test/buss-perry-aggression-questionnaire

BINGE EATING: https://psychology-tools.com/test/binge-eating-scale

EATING DISORDER: https://psychology-tools.com/test/eat-26

INTERNET/PHONE: https://psychology-tools.com/test/internet-addiction-assessment

SEXUALLY COMPULSIVE: https://psychology-tools.com/test/sast

PORN ADDICTION: https://pornaddictiontest.com/test/ *

*The porn addiction is an interesting aspect of addiction study as, like sexual and intimate (online teasing without meeting) infidelity, the damage strongly impacts the significant other as much, or more, than the person engaging in the activity. On the following page you will see the different hormones that impact lust, versus attraction and attachment.

If your intimate partner relationship is at risk or has been damaged by any level of infidelity, then we suggest you further research Dr. Kevin Skinner's work (creator of the porn addict test above). Dr. Skinner is an authority on sexually compulsive behavior, infidelity, and trauma from sexual betrayal. He is a faculty member of IITAP (International Institute of Trauma and Addiction Professionals) and Clinical Director and Co-Founder of Addo Recovery. In addition, he's the Clinical Director and Co-Founder of Bloom for Women, a global online community of women with sexual trauma. Over the last 15 years, his research investigates how sexual betrayal creates PTSD-like symptoms in the betrayed spouse.

His website has tests and help for both people involved in sexual and intimacy behavior pursuits and the significant other impacted. Here is the link for his website for more information:

https://www.discoverandchange.com/tests/

There are apps as well as recovery groups that can help you achieve your recovery goals. Sober Tool, is an example of an app developed by a certified drug and alcohol counselor that focuses on preventing a person in recovery from relapsing. Some of the materials the app includes are related to mindfulness training, a 12-step practice to sobriety, stress reduction techniques and more.

SELF ACCEPTANCE

Achieving sobriety and entering recovery is a tremendous accomplishment. Your family, peers, and friends will likely wish to celebrate milestones along the recovery path. This may challenge your emotional comfort if it reminds you of the negative impact your addiction had on those you care for. Feelings of guilt, shame, and stress may instigate self-deprecating thoughts that will have to be quashed with a vengeance. Self-forgiveness in recovery is critical to maintain your focus on a better tomorrow. If you struggle with worthiness or self-forgiveness, find a counselor or chaplain to help you through this personal challenge and keep you on your recovery track.

SELF-CARE IN RECOVERY INCLUDES:

- Self-compassion, which is the root of forgiveness. It isn't about making excuses, but rather recognizing the trauma events and experiences that led you to self-harming coping behaviors. Self-compassion provides you're the foundation to recognize you are no longer defined by your past actions or behaviors and keeps your focus on new wellness

- Earning forgiveness may be a challenge as others may take time or refuse to forgive you. You cannot control their response, you can only focus on taking responsibility for your past actions, genuinely apologize, and be consistent in your words and actions for an improved future relationship. You may not find this easy, especially if you cannot forgive yourself first.

- Self-flagellation does not move you forward so giving yourself grace and understanding that no one is perfect, and we all have moments of unhealthy and unbeneficial actions and behaviors is a good starting point. While it is good to view your recovery self with high moral standards make sure they are realistic and provide you time to build new habits and actions to manage your triggers and attain planned goals.

- You cannot change your past so accept it as a lesson to reflect and study on. Ensure your new goals and habits are documented so you can see your progress and admire your efforts.
    - Recognize that you are not the same person that you were so you cannot see yourself in that light anymore. The most emotionally intelligent among us are all a work of continual improvement.
- Create a physical ritual with emotional attachment, like daily journaling, gratefulness exercises, prayer, or meditation. A ritual brings about inner peace which can help bring closure to your old self and pave the way to self-forgiveness

Self-acceptance and forgiveness will take time. Give yourself grace and kudos for every action accomplished as you move forward in wellness.

What insights did the quizzes provide you that you didn't consider prior to taking them?

____

____

____

____

HORMONE HIJACKING - SURVIVE THE SNEAKEST EMEMY - OUR BRAIN!

Emotion is the word we use to describe feelings. Many scientific books and articles relate emotions to simple chemical reactions. While emotions are the sensory responses to chemicals released in the bloodstream, they are also electrically charged, sending out 'vibes' to those around us, our resonance. To truly understand how the mental ambush impacts us, ***Going Beyond the Call*** focuses on the neuroscience underlying trauma response and not just the typical psychological first aid and critical incident response. When our entire physiology is impacted, true mental fitness needs to include a logical understanding of how our mind, body, and relationships (with self and others) intertwine. With this clarity, the cognitive center of our brain has the right information to lead the charge on lasting changes and prevent long term illness and avoid costly escalated human interactions.

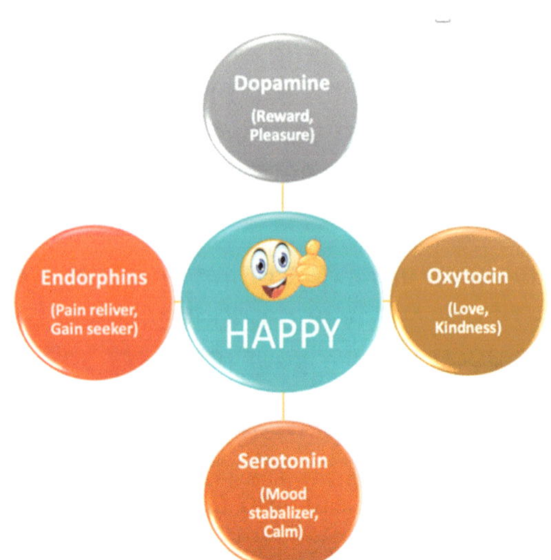

DOPAMINE: Pleasure, motivation, learning

OXYTOCIN: Trust, relationships, love

SEROTONIN: Acceptance of self and others, feelings of calm, significance

ENDORPHINS: Brief euphoria response to pain and stress.

In her book, ***Molecules of Emotion*** Dr. Candace Pert, writes about the physics of emotion and how the chemical signals, a mixture of peptides, have far reaching effects *"as our feelings change, this mixture of peptides travels throughout your body and your brain. And they're literally changing the chemistry of every cell in your body – and sending out vibrations to other people. We're not just little hunks of meat. We're vibrating like a tuning fork — we send out a vibration to other people. We broadcast and receive. Thus, the emotions orchestrate the interactions among all our organs and systems to control that."*

Hormones are also significantly impacted by your environment, relationships, diet, exercise regime, and, in some cases, as well as your gut. Many are unaware that your gut bacteria produce and react to the same neurochemicals as the brain to regulate mood and cognitive abilities.

WATCH: https://youtu.be/B9RruLkAUm8 Your Gut Microbiome: The Most Important Organ You've Never Heard Of | Erika Ebbel Angle | TEDxFargo and https://youtu.be/awtmTJW9ic8 Food for thought: How your belly controls your brain | Ruairi Robertson

*Dopamine makes our brains do dumb-ass things! **WATCH:** Addiction Neuroscience 101 https://youtu.be/bwZcPwlRRcc*

Why do alcohol, opioid, and other drugs have such compelling control over our decision making. This will help us understand our craving challenges as well as help us see those we serve in a more educated light. It also shares how medication can help our behavioral control.

Take-away: How I will see others as well as myself when it comes to dopamine hijacking:

____

____

Oxytocin

This Harvard link shares how a team of scientists led by Dr. Helen Fisher at Rutgers, show where hormones come into play for lust, attraction, and attachment. Too much oxytocin can lead to a not so helpful outcome. Sexual arousal (but not necessarily attachment) appears to turn off regions in our brain that regulate critical thinking, self-awareness, and rational behavior, including parts of the prefrontal cortex.

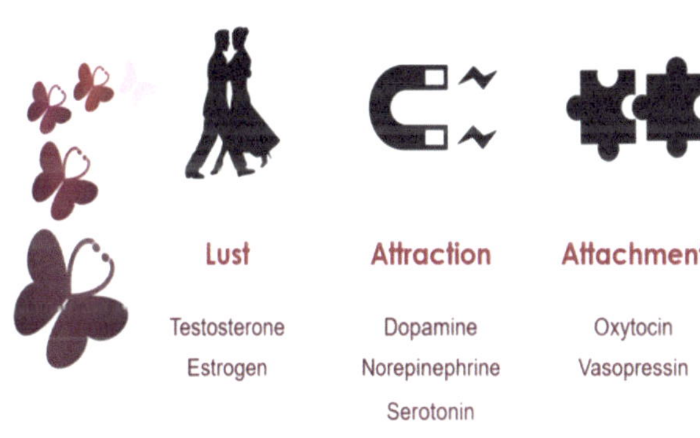

Table 1: Love can be distilled into three categories: lust, attraction, and attachment. Though there are overlaps and subtleties to each, each type is characterized by its own set of hormones. Testosterone and estrogen drive lust; dopamine, norepinephrine, and serotonin create attraction; and oxytocin and vasopressin mediate attachment.

https://sitn.hms.harvard.edu/flash/2017/love-actually-science-behind-lust-attraction-companionship/

Have you ever done something regrettable in lust or love?

____

____

____

____

***Serotonin:* This inhibitory neurotransmitter plays a vital role in mood regulation.**

We have two very important and positive emotions we like to chase, pleasure and happiness. Some believe these emotions are the same however neuroscience looks at it a differently. In the book, ***"Hacking of the American Mind,"*** author Dr. Robert Lustig provides seven differences between pleasure and happiness that will redefine how we look our feel-good pursuits.

1. Pleasure is visceral; happiness is ethereal.
2. Pleasure is short-lived; happiness is long-lived.
3. Pleasure is taking; happiness is giving.
4. Pleasure can be achieved with substances; happiness cannot be achieved with substances.
5. Pleasure can be experienced alone; happiness is usually experienced in social groups.
6. Extremes of pleasure all lead to addiction, whether they be substances or behaviors. There's no such thing as being addicted to too much happiness.
7. Pleasure is dopamine; happiness is serotonin.

Let's go back to your gut. Research has found that the overwhelming amount of serotonin in your body, estimated at ninety-five percent is produced in the lining of your gastrointestinal (GI) tract with the remaining produced by the brain, this is called the gut-brain axis. Gut bacteria produce hundreds of neurochemicals, and our brains use these to regulate basic physiological processes and mental processes including, learning, memory, and mood. It also responds to the same neurochemicals, such as GABA, serotonin, norepinephrine, dopamine, acetylcholine, and melatonin our brains use to regulate mood and cognition. Research has shown that Lactobacillus, or probiotics improved mood in mice (https://www.apa.org/monitor/2012/09/gut-feeling) and research is ongoing to make the gut-brain connection. For emerging or mild symptoms, it may be worth taking a daily supplement or probiotic or prebiotic/probiotic mix, check with your doctor first. (https://www.ncbi.nlm.nih.gov/pmc/articles/PMC7510518/)

Poor serotonin regulation can cause a myriad of symptoms that we may not immediately associate to a low chemical in our brain: mood disorders, such as depression, anxiety, and some research indicating it is prevalent in obsessive-compulsive disorder and anger management issues as examples. If your body is not regulating serotonin well, then your outlook on life may be grim. Most cases of serotonin deficiency are idiopathic, meaning doctors are unable to find a specific cause via a test, so they diagnose based on behavioral symptoms. Psychiatrists and physicians routinely prescribe selective serotonin reuptake inhibitors (SSRI's) to help regulate people with depression and anxiety. However, not all mood disorders are caused by serotonin regulation, so these medications do not work for everyone. If you have found SSRI's to be unhelpful, don't give up; push your medical advisory team to seek other answers. Medication on its own will also not magically fix any underlying trauma, however it may improve your mental wellness enough that you can focus on therapy goals and gain back your mental fitness.

Some genetic dispositions may also affect the body's ability to make or metabolize serotonin, in which case medication may provide more lasting help. Other factors like lifestyle; hormonal shifts (natural or person altered); menopause; pregnancy; aging; lack of sunlight; chronic stress; poor nutrition; and as above, certain drugs, also impact your serotonin regulation. Happiness, peace, and joy are the goal in life, so researching, reaching out, and accepting medication and therapy options to optimize your mental fitness are worth trying.

LOW SEROTONIN SIGNS AND SYMPTOMS

Depression	Circadian rhythm (sleep)dysfunction	Challenges with deep REM sleep	Appetite Issues Over/under eating	Memory or Learning challenges
Anxiety	Chronic Pain	ADD/ADHD	Dementia (early warning)	Schizophrenia

Has learning about serotonin regulation changed how I feel about medication and lifestyle modifications? What are you willing to try?

____

____

____

Endorphin: Combination of two compounds, endogenous and morphine

Endorphins are a happy chemical but work in two ways by providing a burst of euphoria as it reduces pain and discomfort. Endorphins are our body's natural morphine. The higher the level of endorphin release, the lower the pain we feel and the more relaxed, even euphoric, we can become. This provides a natural high in our brains that will encourage repeated experience, which is why some drugs can become addictive so fast.

What are some of the healthy experiences, supplements, and foods that can provide a more natural high? Some of the following list is subjective as research has been done on animals and not definitive on humans. These suggestions may release endorphins, activate opioid receptors, and re-sensitize the brain after addiction. Review with your doctor for the right fit for you.

High intensity exercise	Sleep with 4-5 distinct REM cycles	Minimum of 10 minutes of sun/day	Social interaction (that you like)	Cold therapy
Massage	Magnesium	Melatonin for sleep	Healthy meal prep/ mindful eating	Dark Chocolate (in moderation)
Butyrate 150–300 mg/day	Capsaicin / Chili or other spicy food	Safe and loving sexual intercourse	Creative pursuits, music, dance, art	Time with good friends

What are you willing to try to naturally boost your happy brain chemicals?

____

____

LONG TERM STRESS: **How stress affects your brain - Madhumita Murgia**
Watch: https://youtu.be/WuyPuH9ojCE

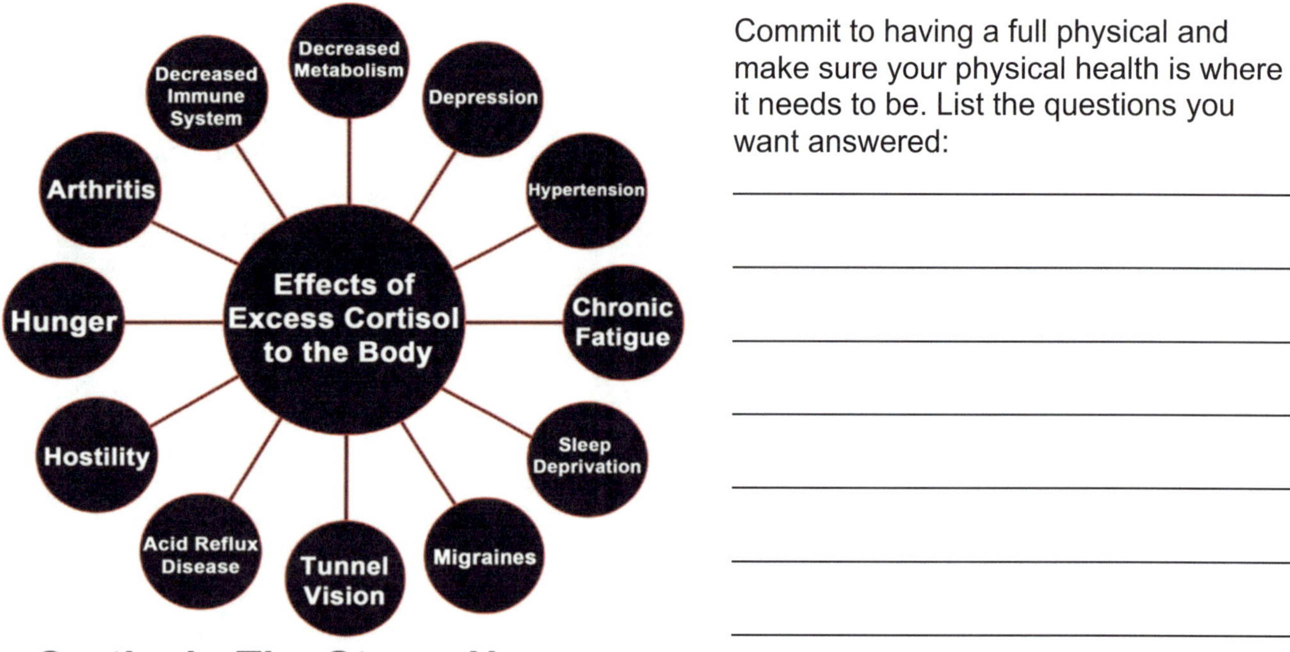

Cortisol - The Stress Hormone

Commit to having a full physical and make sure your physical health is where it needs to be. List the questions you want answered:

____

____

____

____

____

____

____

A TIME FOR THERAPY

Now we have a little broader understanding of how our own brain can ambush our mental fitness without proper self-management. There are a lot of healthy options to release our happy chemicals, however, remember the impact of substance and behavior addictions will have a higher release of chemicals than healthier pursuits. Full recovery from a very unbalanced chemical system may take extra effort and significant time before you are satisfied with your happy chemical balance. Being aware and mindful of the impact of our internal maladaptive systems allow for more curiosity to find the right solution that is best for you.

More imbalance recovery options are listed below. If one treatment option, or provider, doesn't work for you please don't quit, mental fitness is not an overnight fix. There are many types of therapy and providers. In person and online therapy options are plentiful and the right fit for you may take a little investigation. We suggest you seek out a service that is specifically trained in your discipline or at minimum, first responder or military specific. They will be more aware of the specialized trauma impacts of managing the unmanageable on a regular basis. We have suggested a few at the back of our book: GBTCbook.com

We also suggest a confidential discussion with your local Chaplain, most who have been trained in first responder counseling. They are trained as non-denomination sources and have the unique ability to discuss suicidality with a broader "duty of care" window to make it safer for you to talk about this critical issue.

Cognitive Behavioral Therapy (CBT)	Twelve-step facilitation therapy ("12-step programs")	Rational Emotive Behavior Therapy (REBT)	One-On-One And Family Counseling
Treatment with Medication, Pharmacological	Dialectical Behavioral Therapy (DBT)	Group Therapy and Support Groups	Experiential Therapy (Rope courses, music, art)
Biofeedback And EMDR	Contingency Management (CM)	Trauma affect regulation	Equine And Animal Therapy
Nicotinamide Adenine Dinucleotide NAD + Therapy	Hypnotherapy	Self-care behavior and lifestyle management	Motivational Interviewing

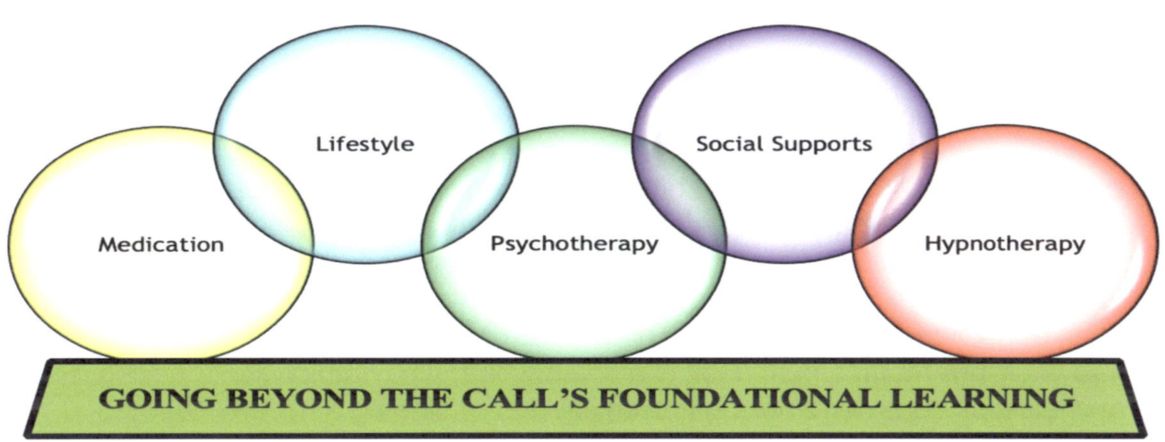

DEVELOPING MENTAL FITNESS

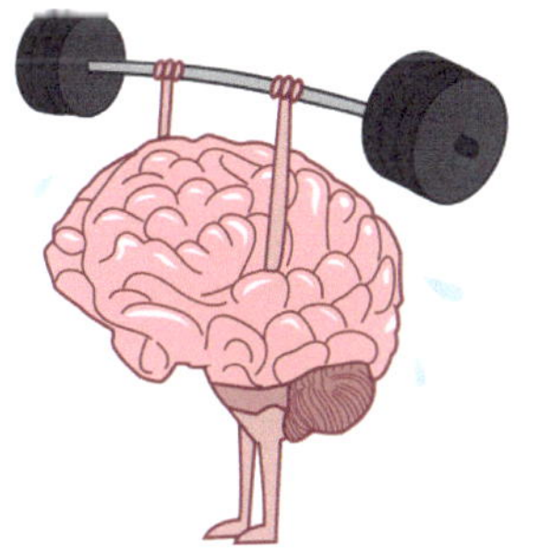

BRAIN PLASTICITY:
WATCH: https://youtu.be/ELpfYCZa87g

Neuroplasticity includes several different processes taking place throughout a lifetime.

The environment plays a key role in influencing plasticity. In addition to genetic factors, the brain is shaped by the characteristics of a person's environment and by the actions of that same person. Gray matter can shrink or thicken; neural connections can be forged and refined or weakened and severed. Changes in the physical brain manifest as changes in how we think or act, basically our habits. The saying “we are what we think,” needs to become our mantra for healthy mental fitness.

The general assumption that all you need is 21 days, this came from the book Psycho-Cybernetics by Maxwell Maltz, a plastic surgeon explaining to his patients how long it would take to get used to their new face. More studied research indicates this isn't the average or even the case for many. So, if you have been frustrated when after a month something hasn't "stuck," know you are not alone. The new consensus is individuals varied from 18 days to 254 days, with the average coming in at 66 days. The most amazing thing about our brain is, with a sustained and focused effort, it can change and develop new ways of thinking and doing that improve our overall health and relationships regardless of your starting point. Just remember, as the video shows, when we engage in new habits, those old pathways are still there; give yourself grace in understanding it will take time for that old pathway to shrink.

Going Beyond the Call's hashtag #the1stLineOfHealing stems from our belief that with adaptive resiliency, emotional intelligence, and trauma-informed mindfulness, we have the power to change our inner selves and our external relationships for the better. Self-care starts when we understand where we are at and where we want to be in both health and happiness.

To break an old habit, keep these tips in mind:

- It's easier to break an old habit by starting a new one versus just stopping.
- There is no 'set' time that a new habit will take hold. Each one will depend on a mix of circumstances, personality, motivation, and the habit or addiction being purged.
- You must do it for you. Habit change will happen faster when it aligns to your own decision and values and not because of an external pressure.
- Ensure your new replacement habit is a healthy one, (i.e., smoking to snacking isn't a great choice, so consider smoking to working out, or starting a healthy hobby).
- The longer the habit or addiction, the longer it will take to shrink that old neural pathway and strengthen your new habit, so give yourself grace and time.
- If your habit is so strong it is addictive, then seeking support and accountability partners will help you achieve your new healthy objective faster and easier.
- New habits are easier to form when we like and love ourselves enough to want to change, so emotional intelligence and resiliency building are important building blocks in order to change.

What habit would you like to alter for a new healthier you? What are you willing to commit to for a minimum of three months?

____

____

____

____

____

____

LOVE THYSELF

Self-love is a continuing process of highs and lows. Your resiliency levels need to adapt to situations and changing circumstances in personal, environmental, and social hardships. The more you focus on your emotional intelligence, the more adaptable you become. For good mental fitness we want to be in a healthy range, but that may not always be true when trauma has us second guessing ourselves. Rather than a right or wrong score here, we want you to pay attention to the extreme highs or lows.

Self-love quiz **Score a number between 1 and 5**	**Rarely to Always 1 - 5**
I feel comfortable in my own skin	
I can let go of my mistakes, forgive myself and move on	
When I look in the mirror, I feel good about myself	
I can laugh at myself when I make a slight error or goofy action	
I believe I am a likeable person to most people	
When I feel sad, I seek positive activities and thoughts to improve my mood	
I handle critical and constructive criticism well and learn from feedback	
I am comfortable with my boundaries and saying “no” when I am tired, stressed, or uninterested in a request someone makes	
I trust myself to make good decisions when my emotions are high	
I am confident I add value to other’s lives	
I am good with my process of weighing decisions and making good choices	
I mostly choose healthy options to feed my mental health and body	
I give myself grace and kindness when things are not going well	
I recognize I am perfectly imperfect and do not accept internal abuse	
After I accomplish something, I reward myself for a job well done	
I believe my voice and opinion matters and express myself assertively	
I am comfortable being fully myself when around family and friends	
I can accept compliments and give thanks when praised	
I am pleased with my contributions in life (family, career, giving back)	
I am happy with my own company	
I am comfortable discussing my feelings with those close to me	
I highly rank self-care and self-soothing activities to build the best version of myself	

Healthy self-love is realistic and encompasses all elements of emotional intelligence. Emotional intelligence or Emotional Quotient (EI or EQ) is your ability to understand and manage your feelings and your ability to self-motivate and self-manage. It also requires active awareness on how others feel and respond to their emotions.

Emotional intelligence can be broken down into five elements: self-awareness, self-regulation, motivation, social skills, and empathy.

In public safety leadership, and with peers, we may come across the narcissist. While we all have a little "all about me" in us, whether overt or discreet, the disorder can cause additional stress in the workplace. It is not only important that boots on the ground have empathy towards the community they serve, but they also need to know whoever is in charge will lead the way. Internal administration is often voiced as an area members have a lack of trust when it comes to seeking help or support.

To become a trauma-informed organization, policy, procedures, and leadership all need to transform the culture first before it becomes mainstream and aids better community relations. Narcissism in leadership bleeds a stigma upon mental fitness and will significantly cost the organization both in risk, safety, and human resource management. At "***Going Beyond the Call***" we help organizations with both their most important asset, their people, and their overall organizational wellness and risk management practices.

By Frits Ahlefeldt

WATCH: Self-love vs narcissism
https://youtu.be/VjFY7SvXWzw

WATCH: Covert Narcissism https://youtu.be/mOdZHi6Z5fY

Take a moment and journal about your perception of self-love after this section. Were you surprised at your result? Would you like to change your result?

____

____

____

____

Do you have a narcissist in your life that negatively influences your self-love result?

____

____

____

____

"We teach ourselves and others how to treat us.
Through internal dialogue, external expressions, and chosen boundaries we can choose to control toxicity within and without."
~ Deirdre von Krauskopf

GETTING TO KNOW ME

How well do you really know yourself? How much time have you spent investigating and discovering what makes you act and react in the world? What traits you admire, or strive for, within yourself?

"Character Strengths and Virtues" was written by Christopher Peterson and Martin Seligman (pioneer of positive psychology). Their concept was to measure the humanist ideas of virtue in a rigorously scientific manner in relation to positive psychology. Their list has six core virtues, with 24 measurable character strengths. In areas of recruitment, promotion, and leadership this basic identification of who we are comes into play repeatedly.

What are your top core virtues and characteristics. Which ones do you believe you should focus on for growth and development?

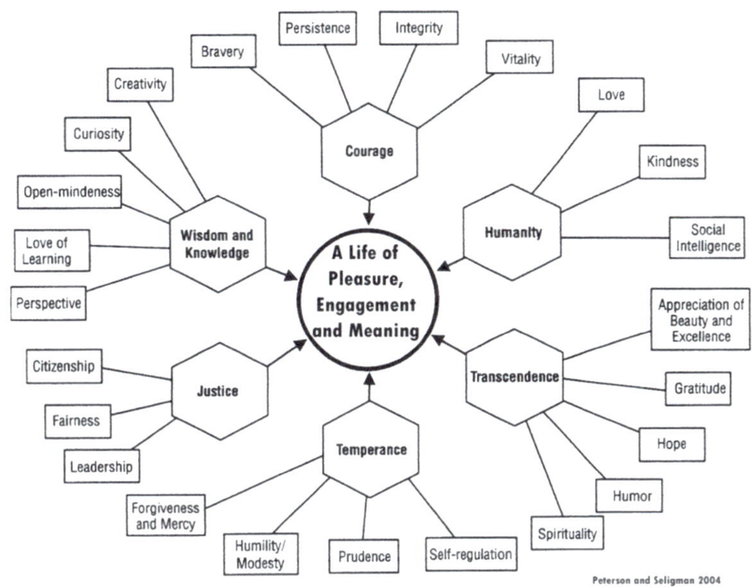

____

____

____

____

Truly knowing our strengths and areas of improvement are invaluable for adaptable resilience and emotional intelligence. We are not great at all things; however, we are capable of change when we self-direct our growth. Through this resiliency building section we will learn that we have very little control over changing other people. Focus is best served in changing ourselves, our reactive responsiveness, and our relationship success strengths for optimum personal health. Through this self-work we gain the skills and mindset to utilize strategic management and influence tactics and tools to lead other to their own best options.

When we haven't spent any time understanding what makes us tick it can be more challenging to build our adaptive resiliency and change our neural pathways to more productive mental fitness.

We can explore our self-determined intelligence by understanding that not all people are meant to follow the same path. Let's start with intelligence. How many of you struggled in school, in certain subjects, or overall? How many heard that famous teacher's line ***"if you only applied yourself, you would do so much better?"*** We have been programmed to believe that our level of intelligence is only derived from one type of measured testing, our intelligence quotient (IQ). The world would fall apart if we were all PhD's in academic pursuits. This skewed view of being smart can lead some to begin a self-defeating internal dialogue at a young age. This negative imprinting can be further lodged in our minds if the adults around you fall into a completely different category.

Anxiety is increasing for many youths as more extracurricular classes and activities are removed from general education. A couple generations ago one may not have done well academically but would have found their place in other classes or activities in school and be known for excelling in that arena. Whether it was art, music, shop, athletics, drama, or the audio/visual club, a person could build friendships and feel competent in a self-motivating pursuit. Without that belief in one's abilities isolation, depression, anxiety, and overall self-love and appreciation may take hold. In Harvard psychologist, Howard Gardner's book ***"Frames of Mind: The Theory of Multiple Intelligences"*** details eight general intelligences and proposes a ninth, "existentialist intelligence." Each can assist someone in understanding where their strengths lay and how to grow where they excel, including how to manage one's career path when options arise.

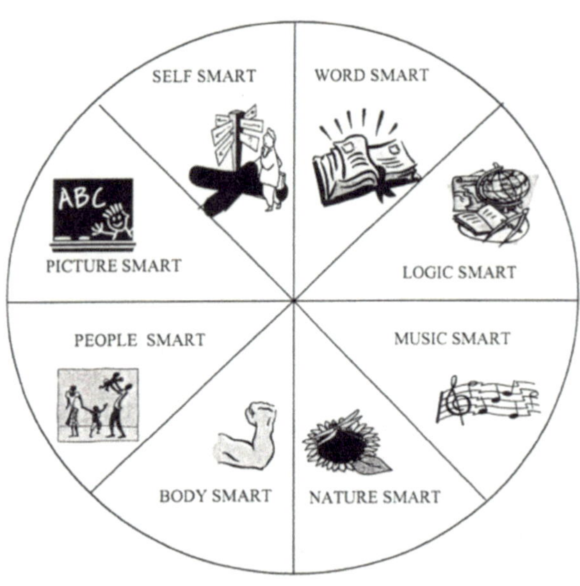

PRIORITIZE YOUR MULTIPLE INTELLIGENCES:

1. ____________________
2. ____________________
3. ____________________
4. ____________________
5. ____________________
6. ____________________
7. ____________________
8. ____________________

Educational curriculum has traditionally taught in an auditory fashion with some visual reference; if you fall in one of the other learning styles you likely struggled in most of your classes. Studies have shown that on average the population falls into this mix: 65% **visual**, 30% **auditory** and 5% **kinesthetic.** If the learning you are immersed in does not have the right style, then it may be up to you to add in the elements that will make new information stick.

Ideally, educators and facilitators will teach in a manner that encompasses all intelligences and all learning styles to broadly encompass each students' strengths. In our 2-day workshops we ensure that we have a good mix of varied listening and visuals, with two instructors engaging the audience, use of PowerPoint plus videos and making exercises interactive and physical. Even this workbook is designed so you look up other materials (in our book), link to videos, and have exercises for the kinesthetic aspect. As we grow, we will have more videos, more audible downloads, and we are working on an interactive podcast to continue to engage our students.

Have you ever considered what your best learning style is and how you can apply that to bettering your personal growth and resiliency? How about your children, family, friends, and peers? If you are a training officer, do you encompass different learning styles into your training?

LEARNING STYLES

Visual Learners	Visual memory and perception	Leans in, watchful, highlights materials, likes doodling, charts, graphs, color coding, catchy visuals
Auditory Learners	Auditory memory and perception	Focus on tone, pitch, volume, in-person, audio, and video preference. Prefer discussion, reading aloud, and dialogue
Read/Write Learners	Tactile recall and perception	Preference for text, rewriting, reviewing written formats
Kinesthetic Learner	Physical memory and perception	Hands on, experiments, demonstrations, will want to stand up or move around while learning
SECONDARY LEARNING STYLE		
Verbal Learning	Auditory-Verbal or Verbal (Linguistic) Style	Books, journals, notes that they will often read aloud, repetitive listening while writing
Logical Learning	Reasoning, logic, facts	Problem solving learning, recognizing patterns, working through solutions
Social Learning	Interaction, peer-to-peer, social media	Communication with others is key to set knowledge, they will like discussions, group projects, interactive verbal aspects
Solitary Learning	Self-taught, self-supervised	Self-motivated, self-managed, tendency to be introverts

What did you find most interesting about this segment? How will it change how you view both you own and other people's learning style?

RESILIENCY IS NOT STATIC; YOU HAVE IT AND IT CAN BE BUILT UPON

The American Psychological Association defines resilience as, *"the process and outcome of successfully adapting to difficult or challenging life experiences, especially through mental, emotional, and behavioral flexibility, and adjustment to external and internal demands. Several factors contribute to how well people adapt to adversities, predominant among them (a) the ways in which individuals view and engage with the world, (b) the availability and quality of social resources, and (c) specific coping strategies. Psychological research demonstrates that the resources and skills associated with more positive adaptation (i.e., greater resilience) can be cultivated and practiced, also called psychological resilience."*

It is an easy presumption to know that those entering a high-stress career come to the job with a higher-than-average resiliency. Nature and nurture will also have significant input into how naturally resilient you are. Heredity also plays a part in generational trauma aspects, so knowing where you stand helps guide both your awareness and drives a strategy for growth. We will work on growing your resiliency throughout this program.

Resilience Questionnaire – Before reaching adulthood indicate the most accurate answer for each statement	Definitely True	Probably True	Probably Not True	Definitely Not True
I believe that my mother loved me when I was little.				
I believe my father loved me when I was little.				
When I was little, other people helped my parents/guardians take care of me and they seemed to love me.				
I've heard that when I was an infant someone in my family enjoyed playing with me, and I enjoyed it too.				
When I was a child, there were relatives in my family who made me feel better if I was sad or worried.				
When I was a child, neighbors or my friend's parents seemed to like me.				
When I was a child, teachers, coaches, youth leaders or ministers were there to help me.				
Someone in my family cared about how I was doing in school.				
My family, neighbors and friends talked often about making our lives better.				
We had rules in our house and were expected to keep them consistently				
When I felt really bad, I could almost always find someone I trusted to talk to.				
As a youth, people noticed that I was capable and could get things done.				
I was independent and a go-getter.				
I believed that life is what you make it.				
Adapted from: Southern Kennebec Healthy Start, Augusta, Maine, February 2013				

How many of these resiliency protections factors do you have?

How many were highly positive?

What, if any, actions have you taken to build your resiliency when the score wasn't that high?

MINDFULNESS

WATCH: YouTube
https://youtu.be/w6T02g5hnT4 and
https://youtu.be/o-kMJBWk9E0

"If you are depressed you are living in the past, if you are anxious, you are living in the future. ~ Lao Tzu

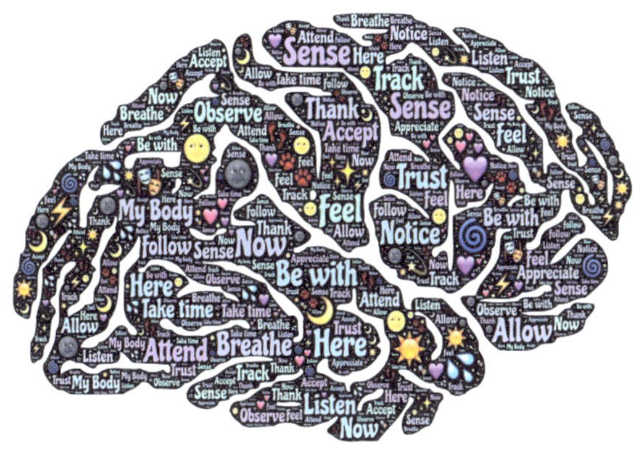

Mindfulness has been defined as "paying attention in a particular way: on purpose, in the present moment in a curious and nonjudgmental way. It is a path to living in peace. A frenzied mind is an overwhelming place to live. Mindfulness focuses our thoughts away from the frenzied drifting that comes from worrying about the past or guessing about the future. When we speed around on an internal superhighway of regret, worry, panic, shame, and fantasy, it is hard to exit from thoughts of "what if's and "shouda/coulda" self-berating. Some may simply avoid the overwhelm and disengage from internal stimuli by zoning out with electronic stimulation that numbs our mind in "other" centered stuff. This too does nothing to bring long-term calm and peace.

Practicing being actively engaged in the here and now, in those moments right in front of us, begins to settle the overwhelm and frenzy. It engages our cognitive ability to begin to break down issues and manage them realistically and purposefully. If past, future, or "other" centered stuff throws us back on that overwhelm superhighway, we can choose to step off again.

There is no fail point in mindfulness, only a commitment to ease the overload of modern living and be present. Learning to recognize our physiological, and psychological triggers, that take us out of the moment helps our self-management, so we are controlling our thoughts versus our thoughts controlling us. With this skill we can better heal internal scars and grow our resiliency.

When your thoughts run amok, do find yourself living in the past or worrying/fantasizing about the future? How does this impact your current quality of life and peace of mind?

____

____

____

COMMUNICATING WITH HUMANS - THE STRUGGLE IS REAL!

(READ: Going Beyond the Call - Chapter 12)

How many times have you been surprised when people do not follow your valuable opinion, or critical direction?

How many times has someone followed another person's direction after they flatly refused yours?

How many times do you feel the person you are interacting with seems like they are ready for a fight before you even speak?

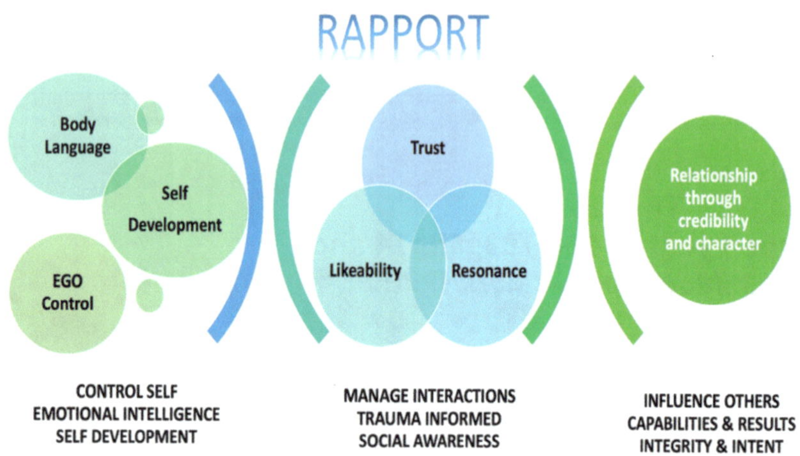

RAPPORT! Is building the authentic elements of words, tone, body language, intent, energy, and presence; all aspects of communication that we bring to every conversation and connection with others. With developed self-control, we can better manage our interactions and influence others. Every stage takes strong emotional intelligence.

There are times when your authority must take precedence; however, 90% of most calls for service do not require this immediately. Almost every call will have a social/emotional element, as you tend to see people during their worst possible moments. Our pre-escalation communication strategy is to manage the best version of you throughout the interaction. Doing so will provide more power to manage and influence the best possible outcome for all involved and avoid escalating and provoking fear, pride, or confusion in others. If the situation calls for escalation, you are well trained to take a more authoritative and command driven approach.

Rapport is not about wanting someone to like you. It's about building a communication bridge so both parties attain the best possible outcome. Avoiding escalation is a good example of why building rapport is important. While de-escalation techniques are critical to have, it will save all involved parties a lot of grief, and paperwork, to avoid escalating to an unknown end. Not only for you and the person(s) you are interacting with, but all those bystanders with their phones recording the moment.

Can you think of a time where, in retrospect, you could have avoided escalation if you had approached the situation differently? Or where another member of your workforce came upon a situation you had under control and created escalation with their words and mannerisms?

____

____

____

COMMUNICATING WITH CALM, SAFE CONFIDENCE

"Your perceptions can have a hold over your emotions and capability to trust yourself. Opening yourself to new ways of thinking, feeling, and reacting provides immense growth and self-reflection. Begin your path to create and project yourself as a calm, safe, confident communicator." ~ Deirdre von Krauskopf

COMMUNICATION BEGINS WITH SELF

SELF- TRUST/PERSONAL COMMITMENT STRENGTHS QUIZ	Rarely	At times	Often	Very Often	Always
Please respond to each statement as it applies to you by entering the corresponding number listed.	**1**	**2**	**3**	**4**	**5**
I make and keep commitments to myself.					
My behavior genuinely reflects my values.					
I am honest and open with others about my wants and needs.					
I am not afraid to take emotional risks or admit my weaknesses.					
I am consistent and predictable in my behaviors and actions.					
People feel safe to confide in me.					
When things do not go as planned, I focus on the lesson, not blaming or mulling on what went wrong.					
My word is my trust bond.					
I hold myself accountable for my actions, choices, and behaviors.					
With new insight or information, I am open to rethinking my ideas.					
When I am wrong, I have no problem apologizing.					
In areas of competence, I have a solid track record of achieving results.					
Total					
Add Totals from each column for total score:					

How did you score?

48 – 60 = Great personal credibility.
36 – 48 = Good you are going in the right direction of self-trust and development.
24 – 36 = Working on your emotional intelligence will boost this score.
Below 24 = Your emotional subconscious has a wee bit too much control. Let's work on this!

Were you surprised by any of the questions or your score? What area(s) do you want to focus on for growth and development?

____

____

____

CONQUERING OVERLOAD AND OVERWHELM

The biggest problem with communications is that we believe the problem is outside ourselves!

One of the challenges you face as public safety professionals is that humans are already overwhelmed. To convey a challenging or difficult message, we want to set our objective, stimulate their interest to co-operate, share intelligence, and chose the most non-confrontational path. In our personal lives we may want to resolve a conflict or engage in a difficult conversation. You may even have practiced what you want to say in your mind and yet you still face the biggest problem in communications today.

When dealing with a heightened emotional situation, the challenge to communication grows significantly. You want to get your ideas through to the other person and most likely their mental cup is already overflowing. That could translate into an agitated encounter, verbal aggressiveness, or their inability to gain emotional or rational perspective. It could also show as a blank stare, or a non-responsive manner. Until a person is ready to hear, you may find yourself wondering, "*why am I even talking*?"

Humans are complicated, over-burdened, and overwhelmed. Until they feel "heard, understood, accepted, respected," they tend to push back, ignore, or repeat themselves. The first job of effective communication in an emotionalized situation is to stimulate their interest. Otherwise, the chances of them receiving your message, as intended, is very low. No wonder there are such communication challenges and quick escalations occurring on the job and at home! We must also admit when our own internal overwhelm and heightened emotions come into play as this is a major aspect of any communication divide.

There is an ancient parable that helps us understand this concept.

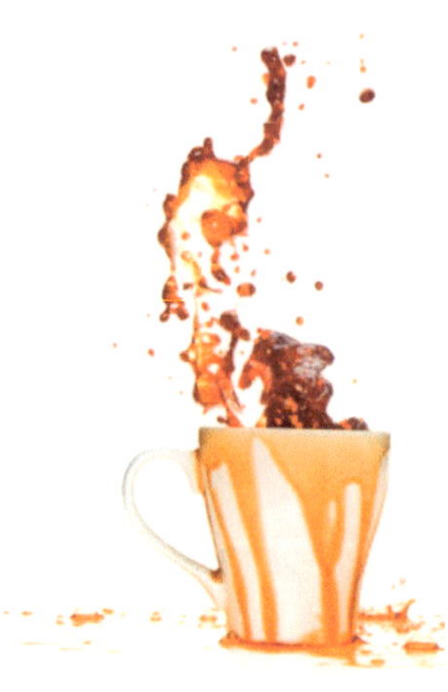

Once, a long time ago, there was a wise Zen master. People from far and near would seek his counsel and ask for his wisdom. Many would come and ask him to teach them, enlighten them. He seldom turned any away.

One day an important man, a man used to command and expecting obedience came to visit the master. "I have come today to ask you to teach me to open my mind to enlightenment."
The tone of the important man's voice was one used to getting his own way. The Zen master smiled and said that they should discuss the matter over a cup of tea.

When the tea was served, the master poured his visitor a cup. He poured, and he poured, and the tea rose to the rim and began to spill over the table and finally spilled onto the clothes of the wealthy man. The visitor jumped up and shouted, "Enough. You are spilling the tea all over. Can't you see the cup is full?"

The master stopped pouring and smiled at his guest. "You are like this teacup, so full that nothing more can be added. Come back to me when the cup is empty. Come back to me with an empty mind."

Think about a time when you realized your mental cup was full and you were not actively engaged in an important conversation. How was the outcome of that communication?

____

____

____

____

Ways to empty our mental cup:

1. Write it down – it releases thoughts from active rumination
2. Talk it out – the act of discussion also helps avoid rumination
3. Pray or meditate – calming the mind helps perspective thinking
4. Digital detox – unplugging from electronics gives your brain a rest
5. Positive distraction – music, workout, pets, hobbies alter your focus

When it is safe and appropriate to do so, building bridges through rapport and strategic communication helps us gain our conversational objective and avoids escalation.

Building rapport in these moments becomes very strategic and intentional. We are going to engage people in the conversation by making sure their cup is emptied so we can stimulate their interest. We will present ourselves in a calm, confident and safe manner to avoid triggering someone in a heightened social/emotional situation. By reading the chapters on communications you will have questioning tactics that help you move the communication forward even with the most challenging conversations.

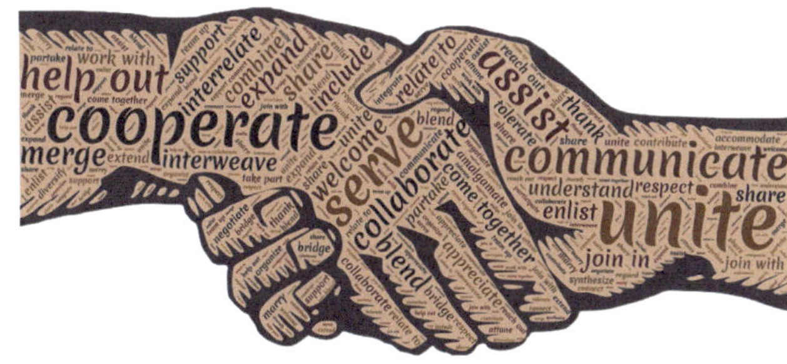

"Between stimulus and response, there is a space. In that space is our power to choose our response. In our response lies our growth and freedom."

~ Viktor Frankl, author of Man's Search for Meaning

Do you see the potential benefit in having a "pre- escalation" mindset for a portion of your on-duty and off-duty conversations? For your time, effort, and to get your message through as intended, does allowing someone to empty their cup makes sense? Does adapting mindful habits to ensure your cup is not inadvertently overflowing make sense?

____

____

____

OVERWHELM IMPACTS BRAIN HEALTH

- **The brain loses ability to engage in critical thinking and problem solving**
- **Situational awareness is diminished**
- **When reaching critical mass, we shut down and if we try to force through, we tend to get sick**
- **Conflict adds to overwhelm, so seek ways to lessen it**

Pre-escalation is the powerful path to peace, so long as peace is an option

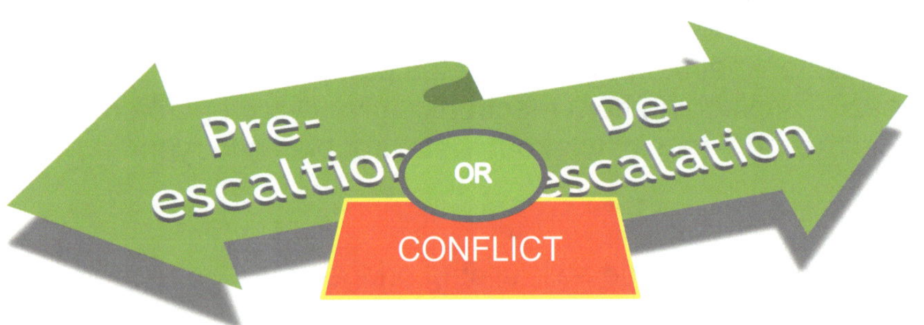

EMOTIONAL AGITATION

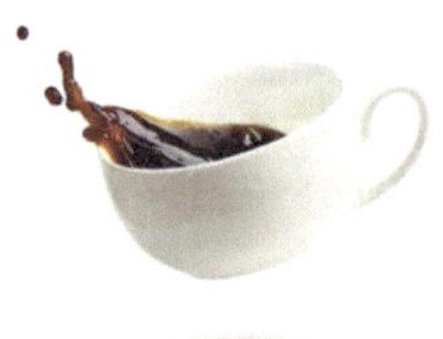

What is inside us spills out when agitated. Picture a brimming coffee cup being walked to a table. Someone bumps the carrier's elbow and what happens? Coffee spills out and wets, or potentially burns the carrier.

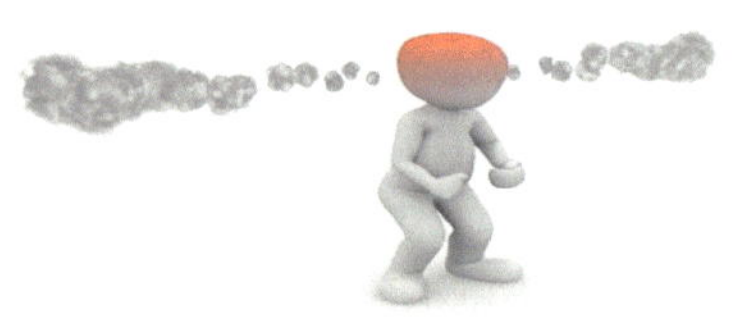

How many times has someone verbally agitated your elbow when your internal hot mess was close to overflowing?

____

____

____

____

What was the trigger or issue that was the tipping point of your overflow and how did you react or likely, overreact?

____

____

____

____

What's in your cup now? What are some common ruminating thoughts that take up your brain space and focus?

____

____

____

____

VERBAL AIKIDO*

Read Chapter 13 ******The following lessons are taken from a licensed program where Sean is a licensed business partner and Deirdre is a global partner with licensed rights to use and adapt this content in these programs and books.*

"Masakatsu Agatsu which means "the true victory is victory over oneself."

The martial art Aikido is often referred to philosophically as a meditation in motion due to the heightened awareness learned in training. All martial arts required mindful concentration; Aikido also includes an empathetic aspect providing a spiritual awareness.

Aikido's founder, Morihei Ueshiba had a spiritual awakening from which he instilled the goal of the warrior was not to kill and destroy; it was to prevent slaughter with a self-developed way of harmony. Aikido tactics are meant to neutralize and control attackers with harmony in a moving meditation; being purposefully aware of both technique and others as you maintain balance.

Going Beyond the Call aligned the spirit of Aikido to our resiliency building, self-control, and communications strategy. Often, we do not consider our tactical advantage when interacting with others. Learning controlled communication is a cornerstone of our pre-escalation mindset. When safe to do so, controlling a situation to avoid de-escalation is a much better option.

Have you ever had a moment in a conversation or while playing a sport where you just 'locked on and zoned into the moment?' What did that feel like?

____

____

____

____

These moments where we feel smarter, sharper than ever, and everything went seamlessly are often call being "in the zone." The Aikido philosophy would say you achieved Ki. When you put all three together, Aikido means: The powerful path to peace. For the public safety professional, this is adapted this to say, *"The powerful path to peace, so long as peace is an option."* When practiced, this philosophy communicates to others that *"in my presence, we are safe. In my presence, we can handle anything. In my presence, we will not be striving for a victor/victim outcome."*

Aikido's principles focus on a centered response, utilization of energy, and nonresistant leading which have a great alignment to nonphysical conflict, verbal attacks, and interpersonal conflict. That is why Aikido is fundamentally distinct from the other martial arts.

Jot down a couple of verbal conflict scenarios that left you angry, frustrated, and ready to battle. You will refer to these in the next couple of pages.

____

____

____

____

____

____

____

____

MANAGING STIMULUS AND RESPONSE WITH A MARTIAL ARTS PHILOSOPHY

Watching the Aikido Masters practice is not what you would expect for a fighting art. You will not see an adversarial battle between aggressor and defender. It is more like two people having a physical exchange where they are giving and receiving energy. With the swirling and flowing movement, it appears more like power dancing than combative posturing.

As an attack comes, the defender does not step in to strike back or block the force of the attack. Instead, the defender accepts the incoming energy and shifts slightly from the line of attack with intent to unite with the attacker's power. Meeting the attacker where they are at, the defender controls the direction of the connection and uses that momentum in their physical response. The underlying principle of Aikido does not resist an attack; instead, those practiced in Aikido learn to blend, control, and redirect the incoming attack of their counterpart. In other words, as Morihei Ueshiba, Founder of Aikido is quoted in the book *The Spirit of Aikido (Ueshiba, Kisshomaru. Spirit of Aikido. Kodansha International, 2013)* as saying; *"A good stance and posture reflect a proper state of mind."*

Let's break down common communication conflict styles with an Aikido perspective. This will help remove all excuses about how you had to exert authority due to the job. For these upcoming exercises use personal relationship examples with someone who means, or meant, a lot to you.

1 PUSH/PUSH FIGHTING STYLE = WIN/LOSE COMMUNICATIONS

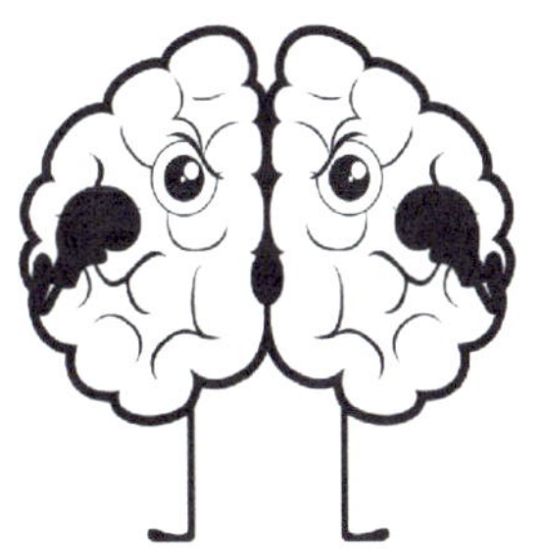

Traditional boxing is where the goal is to hit hard while deflecting the hits of another. Consider how many verbal altercations and arguments follow this formula. The need to win through a position of righteousness, regardless of the damage inflicted along the way. Some are so stuck on winning that every discussion has a hit-block-hit-repeat pattern.

Think about an argument you've had with someone you cared for deeply that had a push-push dynamic and you won. Did you enhance the relationship with the outcome?

____

____

Did you replay the conversation in your mind and wonder whether you could have handled it better?

____

____

2 PUSH/PULL FIGHTING STYLE = WIN/LOSE COMMUNICATIONS

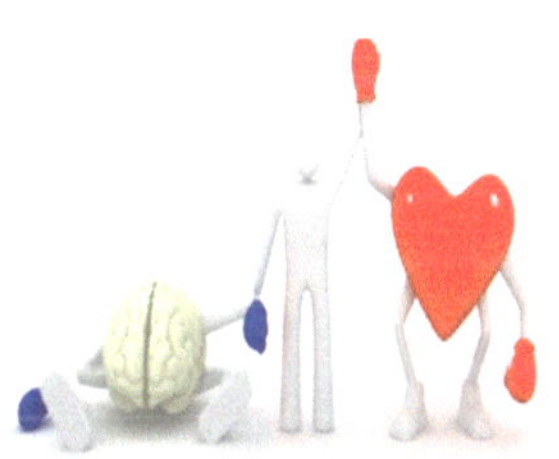

In traditional martial arts the goal is to strike hard using another's weakness, or lesser status against them. You escalate the force through a skillful display of techniques intent on winning at all costs. In communications we can see this in nasty, critical exchanges, sniper-like sarcasm and talking down to another, as well as taking control and dismissing another. One person's skill, aggressiveness, or authority is far superior to another's, and a clear winner takes all outcome ensues, no matter how much damage was done.

With public safety professionals this style of communication would be necessary when safety was paramount to the situation. Your authority and need to control the situation would be reasonable to maintain safety and security for everyone involved. Now consider a conversation where someone you cared for frustrated your emotional balance by bringing up past wrongs, demeaning you, tearing you down in a nasty manner, "putting you in your place."

How did you feel about them after? How many times did you brain regurgitate the conversation? How did that make you feel?

____

____

____

VERBAL AIKIDO IS RESPECTING THE ENERGY, REDIRECTING THE ENERGY, WHILE MAINTAINING BALANCE. THE VERBAL EQUIVILENT TO "I'M NOT FIGHTING; YOU ARE!"

Verbal Aikido is for all the social/emotional interactions where safety is not an immediate risk factor. This is the tactic to use to build rapport, gain co-operation and avoid escalation from your own verbal and physical presence.

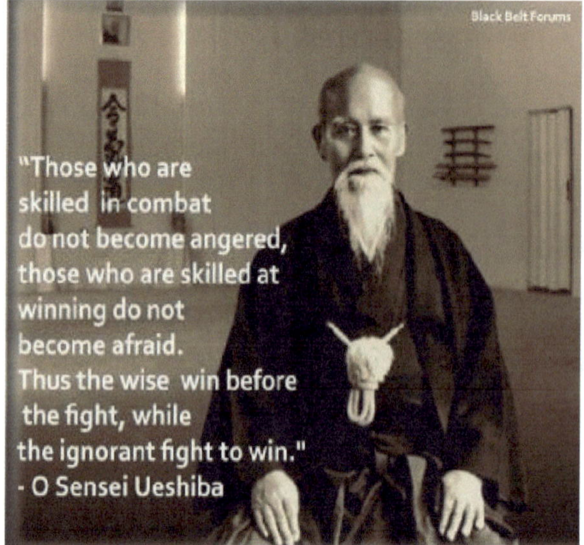

For personal relationships this style will avoid the heated battles and help calm an inflamed topic of discussion. By using this pre-escalation tactic, you are avoiding further emotional escalation without getting pulled into an emotionally triggered response.

The goal is to maintain balance internally while managing and influencing the verbal exchange for the best possible outcome for all involved.

In this difficult communication fight style, the one being attacked is coming from a position of superior strength and their intent to diffuse and calm the aggressor. This approach resolves the dispute faster and achieves the best possible outcome for both sides.

- You don't want to be in front of the energy
- You don't want any push or pull
- You don't want to be in the way of their power
- You don't want to against the energy

- You want to get out of the way of the aggression and stay balanced and grounded!

In communications this would show as a calm, safe, confident presence. To meet them where they are at by acknowledging the aggressor's upset. Maintaining open body language (but readied for escalation if necessary). Empathetic listening and paraphrasing to ensure understanding. Using questioning techniques to redirect emotion to responses requiring logical thinking patterns. Maintaining a caring but focused attention on the outcome objective of the conversation. In a personal setting it may include setting the stage by finding agreement on timing for a difficult conversation. It also may include putting a halt to the moment and agreeing to a pause due to emotion taking over an effective outcome.

Dr. Bessel van der Kolk, author of The Body Keeps Score notes that, *"The biggest issue for traumatized people is that they don't own themselves anymore. Any loud sound, anybody insulting them, hurting them, saying bad things, can hijack them away from themselves. And so, what we have learned is that what makes you resilient to trauma is to own yourself fully."*

COMMUNICATIONS PSYCHOLOGY

FOR THE CONVERSATIONS THAT MATTER MOST

The primary purpose of communication is _______________. As our communication evolves, we move from simply gaining and giving understanding to the synergistic process of attaining _______________ understanding. For individuals to communicate effectively, they must be _______________ and_______________. This generally occurs when they are _____________ and _______________. If you want open and authentic interactions, you, and your conversational partner must both be able and willing.

WHAT YOUR PARTNER REQUIRES:

People are generally able when they feel _______________, and people are generally willing when they are _______________. People are interested when they perceive the possibility of gain or the avoidance of perceived pain. The manageability of risk is factored by considering their own _______________, the _______________ inherent in the context of the interaction, and their level of _______________.

WHAT YOU REQUIRE:

For you to be an effective communicator, you must be able and willing, and these factors are generally present when you are _______________. You may find that you become motivated naturally when, during the process of preparation, you become clear about your _______________, and how that objective aligns with your _______________, and long-term ambitions. The act of preparation will also serve to allay most concerns you may have relating to the interaction by removing many of the 'unknowns.'

NATURAL ENEMIES OF PRODUCTIVE COMMUNICATION ARE:

_______________, _______________, and _______________.

ANSWER KEY:

Fill in the above and read it out loud.

UNDERSTANDING | MUTUAL | RATIONALLY PRESENT | ABLE & WILLING

SAFE | INTERESTED | MANAGEABLE RISK | PERCEIVED STRENGTH | THREAT | TRUST IN YOU

MOTIVATED | PREPARED | INTERACTIVE OBJECTIVE | GOALS

FEAR | PRIDE | CONFUSION

GAINING CONTROL THROUGH SELF-PERSPECTIVE

(Read: Chapters 10, 13, 16, 18, and 19)

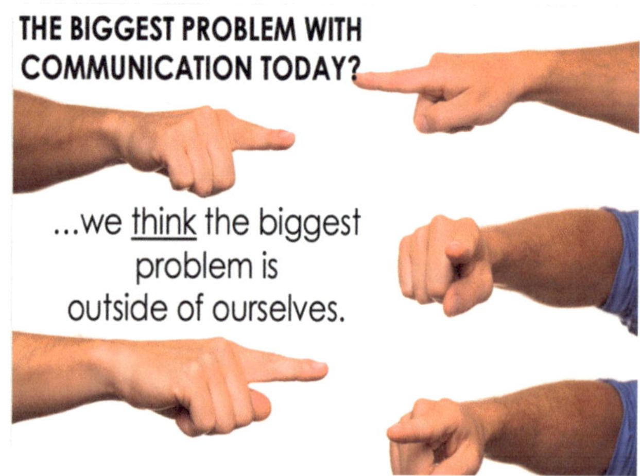

To become the most effective communicators, we want to build our self-control over how we react to situations and learn how to ethically influence others with our actions, body language, and communication skills. Emotions have a large influence on our personality, sense of self, and presentation to the world. They impact our decisions, whether good, bad, big, or small, but emotions do not have to OWN us.

Advances in neuroscience have studied self-control training and can now show us before and after brain scans showing improvements. The results tell us we have the power to change our neurological responses. All of us would like to improve those "knee-jerk" emotional reactions that do not serve us well. Applied training to alter our thinking patterns is possible given our brain's neuroplasticity. Similar to working out to gain muscle mass, when we commit to applying the same repetitive conditioning, we can build our brain's reactionary responses and thus, our behavior.

This workbook will challenge your perceptions, unconscious and conscious bias, outdated beliefs, and self-harming thoughts. We will keep turning to the neuroscience behind repetitive thoughts and actions becoming automated habits and how to change what does not serve a healthy mental fitness. Our goal for you is to systematically create new neural pathways in your brain's communication system and develop a more powerful you!

Once again, we will roll back time and check in on our younger self to fully understand the path that got us were we are today.

What are the top three habits or thinking patterns you wish to change?

___

___

___

Based on input from your family, friends, and significant other, what traits or behaviors have been criticized repeatedly? Where do you think the roots of this trait/behavior comes from, nature or nurture?

___

___

___

WHAT ARE WE MADE OF?

(Read: Chapter 19)

Nature, nurture, personality, emotional intelligence, emotional ego states, and trauma events all combine to make who we are and how we act and react in the world.

Most of us do not spend a lot of time considering or analyzing what makes us whole. The following section will do so and, along with your trauma and resiliency influences from previous sections, you will have a well-rounded understanding of self and what makes you tick!

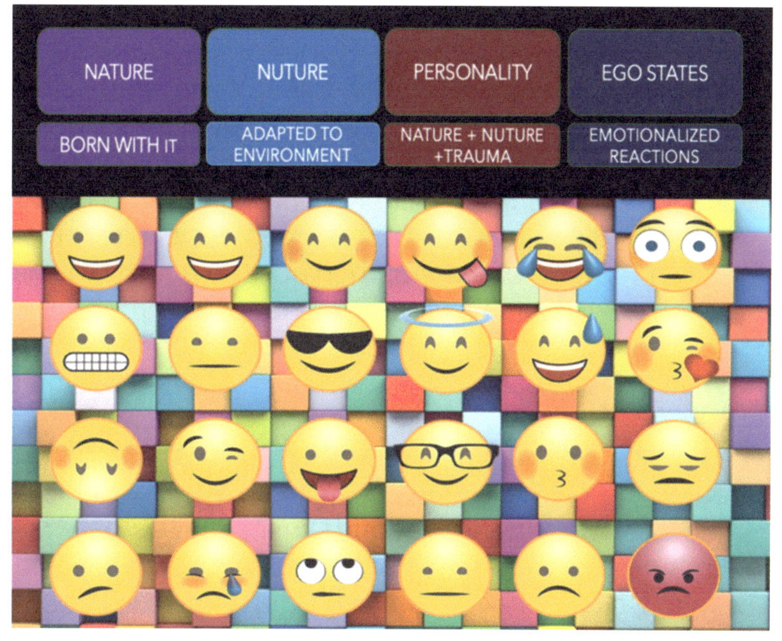

Do you believe you are more a product of nature, or nurture?

____

____

NURTURE:

We discussed ACE's and the power our childhood trauma can have on our developing mind. Environmental, societal, generational, and culture can play a role in our initial behavioral design as well. We will come back to how these further influences how we act and react in the world.

What is your ACE score? ________________ (refer to your quiz results)

Based on the nurture elements listed in the chart below, what were some memorable inputs from the adults and environment you grew up in?

NURTURE INPUTS	
GENERATIONAL	
ENVIRONMENTAL	
SOCIETIAL	
CULTURE	

NATURE:

Psychology experts indicate that natural personalities fall into five broad continuums, and within each you land along the trait continuum. There are as follows: openness, conscientiousness, extraversion, agreeableness, and neuroticism. If you have spent any time around children from the same household, you understand nurture is only part of the equation. Each child is influenced from heredity, genes, and their unique self. Nurturing and trauma inputs will sway where someone sits along the personality continuum, but most children (outside of extreme neglect and abuse) will have stable personality traits that remain consistent in everyday interactions throughout their lifetime. Take a free test here: https://bigfive-test.com you can even compare results with your significant other, family, friends, for interesting discussions on differences and alignments.

The concept of personality tests took hold in the 1920's with Dr. William Marston who created the D.I.S.C personality (he also invented the polygraph machine). Many others have since been developed that offer various levels of personal and career development insight. All may assist your personal and career growth and interpersonal relationships. (Meyers-Briggs, Colors, to more fun character likeness versions). My personal favorite for super quick, peer and family insight is the D.O.P.E. Bird Personality (link below). One's personality can be categorized by four major personalities categories, D.O.P.E. =

Dove:	**kind, patient, accommodating**	**Owl:**	**logical, analytical, systematic**
Peacock:	**showy, outgoing, enthusiastic**	**Eagle:**	**firm, bold, direct, decisive**

We all have bits of each, and our work personality can be quite different than our home life one, but generally, we tend to have one or two stronger areas than others. For further insight or team building, take test here: **https://richardstep.com/dope-personality-type-quiz/dope-bird-4-personality-types-test-questions-online-version/** (results are not free)

What types of personality or interactive behavior testing have you done before? How accurate were they and did it change how you interacted with family, friends, or peers?

____

____

***A LARGE CHOICE OF PERSONALITY TESTS FOUND HERE: openpsychometrics.org**

Now as we start to bring it all together, we see why there is such amazing diversity between people. If we could all be categorized into the highs and lows of five dimensions, humans would be so much easier to manage. A secondary aspect of understanding our general personality is comprehending what drives us. What frames our purpose in life? Often, we can start with a couple of questions to initiate this inner push.

When we understand our personality drivers, we can develop more specific (SMART) goals to include motivators that work best for our 'type'. Based on your personality type score, what changes would you make to your immediate and long-term life goals to keep you on track?

____

____

EMOTIONAL INTELLIGENCE – READ: Chapter 18

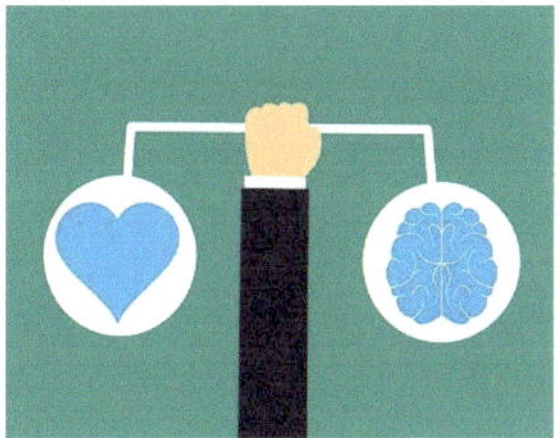

Peter Salovey and John D. Mayer coined the term 'Emotional Intelligence' in 1990 describing it as "a form of social intelligence that involves the ability to monitor one's own and others' feelings and emotions, to discriminate among them, and to use this information to guide one's thinking and action".

Daniel Goleman heard about this research as a science writer for the New York Times and simplified the science into layman's understanding with the book Emotional Intelligence. He worked with David McClelland at Harvard who was among researchers who studied how traditional cognitive intelligence tests didn't do a sufficient job of identifying what it took to be successful in life. Goleman's book shared that emotional intelligence was a far greater indicator of personal and business success in the world. The higher the emotional intelligence, the more successful people became. He described emotionally intelligent people as those with four characteristics:

- Those that understood their own emotions (self-awareness)
- Those that managed their emotions well (self-management)
- Those that remained empathetic to the emotional drives of others (social awareness)
- Those that managed and influenced other's emotions (relationship management)

At ***Going Beyond the Call,*** we believe this science is important as everyday personality tends to change under extreme stress and high emotions. Given many of the events you manage will have one or more emotional or stressed participant, this knowledge becomes a reliable indicator of how a person will act and react in the world.

Not only those you are serving but your own responses and triggers get inflamed during the experience.

The following quiz will give you an idea of where you stand and where you might want to develop.

	RECOGNITION	REGULATION
SELF COMPETENCE	**SELF-AWARENESS** ✓ Self-confidence ✓ Understanding your emotional state ✓ Awareness of your behavior on others ✓ Knowing your emotional reactivity triggers ✓ Accurate self-assessment ✓ Self acceptance ✓ Leaning mindset ✓ Coachable	**SELF-MANAGEMENT** ✓ Adaptive and situational resiliency ✓ Clearly expressing oneself assertively ✓ Utilizing empathy to manage emotional or difficult interactions ✓ Handling conflict effectively with emotional maturity ✓ Problem solving mindset ✓ Self control and discipline ✓ Trustworthiness, Integrity ✓ Role model
SOCIAL COMPETENCE	**SOCIAL AWARENESS** ✓ Situational awareness (reading a room or person) ✓ Social responsibility ✓ Communication savvy ✓ Rapport building skills ✓ Empathetic perspective ✓ Meeting people where they are at ✓ Active and attentive listening skills ✓ Managing bias, social tolerance	**RELATIONSHIP MANAGEMENT** ✓ Managing positive/effective interactions ✓ Accepting and handling conflict ✓ Clearly expressing ideas/information ✓ Sensitive to the emotional reactivity of others, being empathetic ✓ Influencing ethically ✓ Team, collaborative, change, or purpose minded

	Emotional Intelligence Self-Assessment	Never	Rarely	At times	Often	Always
1	I readily admit mistakes and apologize. When I feel angry, I can still stay composed.					
2	I am aware of the physical reactions (twinges, aches, sudden changes) that signal a "gut reaction."					
3	I generally have an accurate idea of how another person perceives me during a particular interaction.					
4	In assessing a situation, I look at my biases and adjust my assessment accordingly.					
5	I can engage in an interaction with another and pretty well size-up that person's mood based on non-verbal signals.					
6	Others feel encouraged after talking to me.					
7	I can keep going on a project, despite obstacles.					
8	I can deal calmly, sensitively, and proactively with the emotional displays of others.					
9	I can identify the emotion I am feeling at any given moment.					
10	I can honestly say how I feel without getting others upset.					
11	I consider my "emotional temperature" before I make important decisions.					
12	I am respected and liked by others, even when they don't agree with me.					
13	I can effectively persuade others to adopt my point of view without coercing them.					
14	When I feel a strong impulse to do something, I usually pause to reflect and decide whether I really want to act on it.					
15	I can effectively persuade others to adopt my point of view without coercing them.					
16	I think about the emotions behind my actions.					
17	I watch how others react to me to understand which of my own behaviors are effective and which are not.					
18	I am good at managing my moods, and I refrain from bringing negative emotions to work.					
19	It's easy to understand why other people feel the way they do.					
20	I can show empathy and match my feelings with those of another person in an interaction.					

Scoring the Tool:
Enter your ratings for each numbered question in the category where it appears. Add the ratings for each category to obtain a total for that specific facet of Emotional Intelligence.

Self-Awareness: 1. ______ 5. ______ 9. ____ 12. ______ 15. ______ TOTAL: _______
Self-Management 3. ______ 6. ______ 10. ____ 13. ______ 18. ______ TOTAL: _______
Social Awareness 4. ______ 7. ______ 14. ____ 17. ______ 19. ______ TOTAL: _______
Relationship Mgt 2. ______ 8. ______ 11. ____ 16. ______ 20. ______ TOTAL: _______

Interpreting Your Score

The range of response is 5 through 25. Any section less that 18 is a good area to do some self-work.

(Adapted from Emily A. Sterrett, Ph. D., in The Manager's Pocket Guide to Emotional Intelligence, 2000, HRD Press: Amherst, MA and from The Handbook of Emotionally Intelligent Leadership by Daniel E. Feldman, 1999, Leadership Performance Solutions)

SELF-AWARENESS - HOW DO YOU PERCEIVE YOU?

Self-awareness is the ability to see ourselves with a studied truth. Very few people take the time to complete a self-inventory. To see who you are, and why you are the person you have become, thus far. Using a separate journal, take the time to review this self-assessment section and create some resilience and emotional intelligence goals. After which you can start to see patterns, behaviors, and ways of being that may or may not serve the person you want to be moving forward.

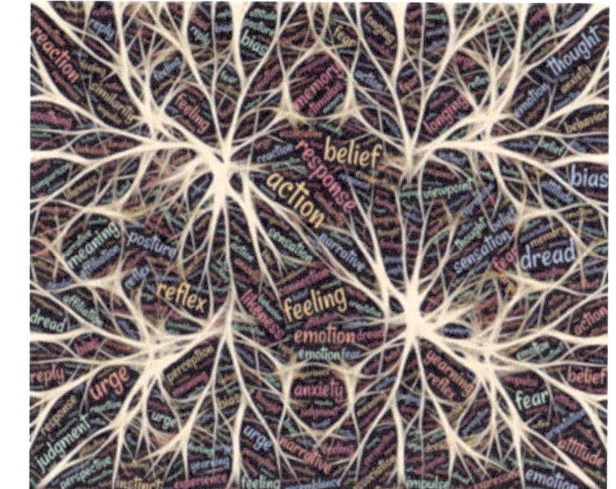

Creating goals is important to achieve our dreams and grow our emotional intelligence; however, without true understanding of who we are to begin with and what motivates us, we can often fail to achieve what makes us happy. When we can recognize what we like about ourselves, we can build on it. When we recognize what we don't like, we can investigate its origins and determine whether that trait or mannerism still serves us well. If not, then we can work on upgrading ourselves.

Self-awareness is broken down by the following aspects:

SELF-ESTEEM: Your opinion on your value as a person.

SELF-IMAGE: How you think others see you.

SELF-CONCEPT: How you see yourself physically, emotionally, socially, and spiritually.

SELF-EFFICACY: Your confidence in your abilities in specific tasks. You may have lower self-confidence in some areas of your life yet high self-efficacy with an area you are really good at.

SELF-PROJECTION: How self-esteem is reflected in the way you treat others. If you Have low self-esteem, you may project this by belittling others. If you have high self-esteem your projection may be very positive.

Let's start with what drives our goals. Drive Theory, created by Clark L. Hull, is based on the principle that humans are born with specific psychological needs and that a negative state of tension is created within this person's mind until the needs have been satisfied. When this need has been satisfied, the mind's state goes back to a level of relaxation and satisfaction.

Circle which motivates you more? Pain or gain?

These motivations show as one of two drivers:

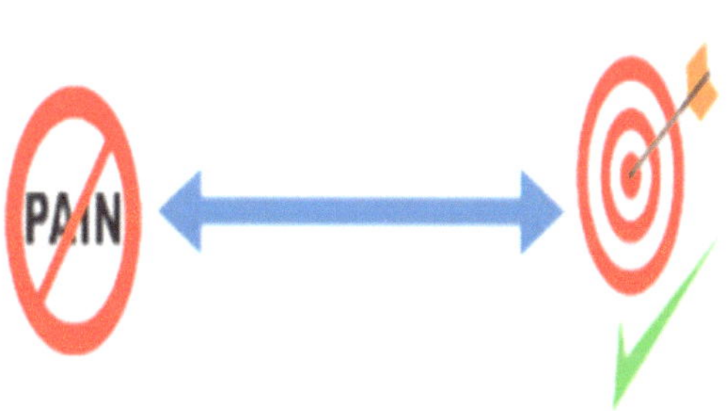

One way is to move towards pleasure, future possibilities, and gain. Having vision and positive planning energizes you.

The other way is to move away from pain, or what you do not want, and you are motivated by problem solving. Negative consequences, looming deadlines, or feeling threatened energize you.

Ideally, we want to work towards having a balance of being motivated by both the positives gains and avoidance of pain, while not letting situations get too problematic before you manage them. The following self-awareness questions will help guide your journaling experience for self-awareness. Use a separate journal for this exercise, as personal writing can be incredibly good for your overall mental health, and it can be very beneficial to notice patterns of thoughts and behaviors. By releasing your thoughts on paper, or computer, you let your brain know you got it down and it can stop reminding you as much. We gave you a few lines to try one or two questions out here.

Questions to explore your personality:

1. Do you feel your personality has changed much since childhood? How so?
2. Which three words best describe you? Would your best friend describe you differently?
3. Does your personality mimic a parent or grandparents?
4. Describe your top 3-5 strengths.
5. Describe your top 3-5 weaknesses. Which one do you want to change the most?
6. What do you admire most about yourself?
7. When making decisions, are you more logic driven, or emotion (gut feeling) driven?
8. What things make you very uncomfortable or scare you? When do you recall that response first manifesting in your childhood?
9. If you could change one negative self-talk that frequents your brain, what would it be? Who said it to you before you said it to yourself?

____

____

____

____

____

____

____

Questions to explore your relationship style

1. Do you treat yourself as you wish others would treat you?
2. Do you treat others as you wish to be treated?
3. Describe the most positively memorable relationship moment you've had.
4. What does the most ideal intimate relationship look like? Do you have it now?
5. On a scale of 1-10, how satisfied are you in your current relationship?
6. What three things would you want to change in your current relationship?
7. What has been the most emotionally devastating moment in any relationship?
8. Who have you loved the deepest? Was it reciprocated? What was it about this love that made it so special?

9. If you only had a few minutes left to live, who would you call? What would you say?
10. If you could tell each parent/guardian exactly how you feel about their style of raising you, what would you say to each? What one thing did you love the most? What one thing did you like the least? Is your parenting style aligned to how you enjoyed or wanted to be parented?

____

____

____

____

____

____

____

____

Self-awareness questions on values and life goals

1. What are the top three life lessons you want instilled in your children, future children, or kids in your circle you may influence?
2. What are your core beliefs, about yourself and others?
3. What are your values and rules? Ways to live by, your 'ought's', 'musts' and 'should do'?
4. How would you describe your ideal 'you'?
5. What life dream did you most have as a child? Did it happen? Or is it still a dream today?
6. What are your top give life goals? On a scale of 1-5, how close are you to achieving each?
7. On a scale of 1-10 how important is each goal? Why?
8. Is there anything that inhibits you from achieving one or more of your goals?
9. If a goal is not possible, have you found a way to get as close to the goal as possible?
10. Based on your earlier exercise about recognizing and growing personal roots, what order of importance would you rank your list?
11. What proportion of time do you dedicate to each of these strengthening roots?
12. What one thing will you commit to doing more of? Describe in detail the commitment to yourself to attain this goal.

____

____

____

____

____

____

SELF-DEFEATING BELIEFS: Listen to David Burns, MD on his podcast

https://feelinggood.com/2018/12/10/118-self-defeating-beliefs-part-1/

What's the difference between Self-Defeating Beliefs (SDBs) vs. Cognitive Distortions?

We discussed Cognitive Distortions earlier, however the difference in a self-defeating belief is that one is tricking your brain to the reality of a situation or thought and can trigger or grow anxiety and depression. You can challenge these types of thoughts and immediately feel better. Whereby, self-defeating beliefs are the internal values you set upon yourself, how you view and compare yourself in the world as a human. They are more ingrained and do not come and go with anxiety, depression, or bad moments; they become part of your self-esteem and self-concept.

Challenging our internal value system takes courage and tenacity to overturn and re-develop newer more thoughtful beliefs based on your current self-work and self-appreciation growth. If you're ingrained a value system that tears you down in a manner you would not subject your family, friends, or others to, then it is time to re-evaluate why you judge yourself with such cruel harshness. Emotional Intelligence includes self-exploration, investigation, and altering aspects of your internal thinking system that often hinders our quality of life.

For full definitions of common self-defeating beliefs CLICK: https://feelinggood.com/wp-content/uploads/2018/11/f1e61-self-defeating-beliefs-list-v-1.pdf

Dr. Burns breaks these down as:

- Achievement: Perfectionism, Perceived perfectionism, and Achievement addiction
- Love: Approval addiction, love addiction, and fear of rejection
- Submissiveness: Pleasing others, conflict phobia, and self-blame
- Demandingness: Other-blame, Entitlement, and Truth
- Depression: Hopelessness, worthlessness, and inferiority
- Anxiety: Emotional perfectionism, anger phobia, emotion phobia, perceived narcissism, brushfire fallacy, spotlight fallacy, magical thinking
- Other: Low frustration tolerance and superman/superwomen expectation

David Burns, MD, provides amazing insight on empowering an improved view of self-development in his book, "**Feeling Great – The Revolutionary New Treatment for Depression and Anxiety.**" If his podcasts resonate with you, I urge you to study his work.

What self-defeating belief(s) do you have?

____

____

____

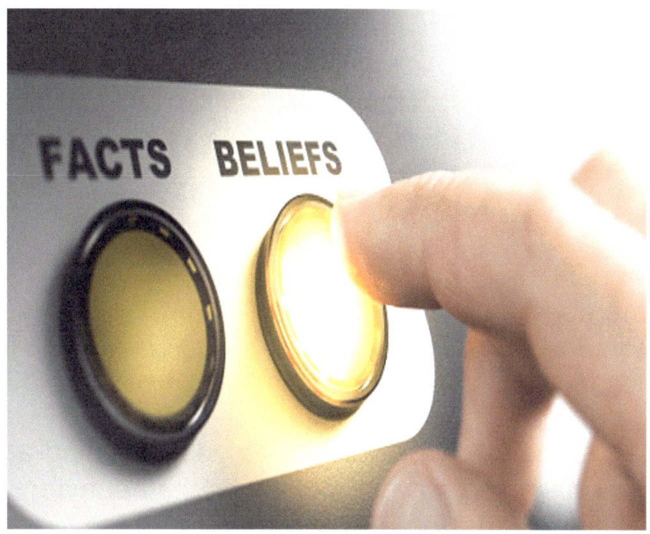

DISEMPOWERING BELIEFS

Other disempowering beliefs are often formed very young and carried into adulthood. That nasty little voice in our head can be quite disturbing and at times, worse than anything another person would say to us, or us to another human. This can lead us to often act as we *think* others see us. In the book, ***"Shakespeare Saved my Life,"*** author, Laura Bates asked death row inmates "*what do your parents think of you being here*?" 100% replied, *'I am exactly where my parents expected me to be'*.

They lived up to the expectations seeded as a belief that they were bad, criminal, destined to die in jail, in their brains from a young age and carried forward unchallenged with their self-image and self-esteem. It can manifest into a little internal bully that limits our happiness and blows up every negative situation unnecessarily.

Your belief system may be allowing the untrained brain crew to steer your ship (cognitive brain) when we really want to Captain our own vessel and navigate our life with updated maps. The Reticular Activating System (RAS) inputs what you feed it. Provide better content and it will seek and attract things that move you towards your goals. Otherwise, your belief system can be an unruly, undisciplined child that is not serving your best interest. A deep dive on self needs good investigative input.

Self-talk is that inner voices that tells us we can or cannot do something. At times we judge ourselves by the worst of comments we heard as children. Never stopping to reassess who we are today, erasing negative chatter that is not serving our mental fitness and grooming what we may want to develop.

A personal inventory may seem like a daunting task, however this self-discovery journey can be eye-opening to who we are and why we are this way. With understanding, we are more apt to make mental fitness changes in our own best interest.

Is your self-talk positive and motivating? If not, do an inventory of the repetitive negative statements that take hold in your brain and assess them.

Negative Self talk statement	Where or when did you first hear these words?	Does the person's opinion who said it matter still?

DISEMPOWERING BELIEFS- COGNITIVE DISSONANCE

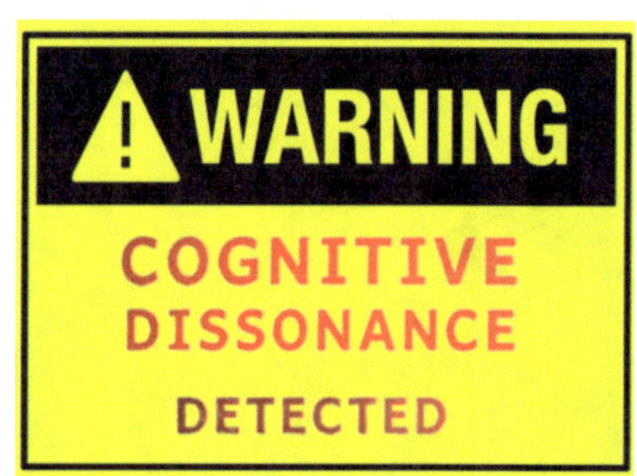

Cognitive dissonance is when our behavior is incongruent with our values, beliefs, or attitudes. It can create tension, discomfort, and, depending on the depth of conflict, it can affect your overall well-being.

It can be caused by a feeling of forced compliance. i.e., a rookie on shift goes along with what senior members do feeling they have no choice but to comply to keep their job.

However, usually our brains will try to ease the discomfort by providing excuses, adopting a new belief to cover the action, or seeking out rationality to convince ourselves the behavior was justified. Our belief is altered but it may cause us conscious or unconscious stress. Some new beliefs or justifications are perfectly acceptable, but many will wear away at our souls. Being honest with ourselves about our excuses can lead to internal healing and put us back on a path aligned with our values, morals, and important core beliefs. See examples below.

WATCH: Cognitive Dissonance/Concepts Unwrapped: https://youtu.be/m_ICO2cBNts

CONDUCT	COGNITIVE BELIEF	UNCOMFORTABLE NEW BELIEF OR JUSTIFICATION
You had a one-night stand affair	Belief you are an honest, honorable person	My spouse doesn't give me enough sexual attention, so I'm justified to seek it elsewhere
You had to take a life in combat	Religious/Moral belief that it is wrong to kill	Killing is acceptable when ordered to do so for God and Country
Your team covers up a wrongdoing to avoid discipline or legal action	Belief that you are law abiding and always do the right thing	This peer is a great guy, they just did a dumb thing. The victim was a bad person anyway

Name something you have a cognitive dissonance with? How have you justified it?

CONDUCT	COGNITIVE BELIEF	UNCOMFORTABLE NEW BELIEF OR JUSTIFICATION

Does the justification sit well with you, or should you do some reflective thinking and forgiveness work with yourself or others?

___

___

How to change:

1) Change the conflicting cognition, attitude, or behavior by adopting a congruent one
2) Acquire new information or supports that outweighs the belief, or
3) Reduce the importance of the conflicting belief

What steps are you willing to take to bring your conduct and belief system back in congruency? (Note, this may not lead to righting a perceived wrong so much as adopting a new way of managing your lifestyle, so you are back to congruency between your actions and cognitive beliefs).

I will heal my cognitive dissonance by doing what?

____

____

____

SELF-ASSESSMENT THROUGH MANY EYES - *Don't take your own word for it*

The Johari window is a tool to look at our own self-assessment and compare it to how others view us. The Johari window involves the open area, hidden area, blind area, and unknown area. This is particularly helpful when you get a 360 perspective from those you know you well. Some responses will be very aligned, and others will be glaringly distant. Knowing how others perceive you can be an honest first step to recognizing our full spectrum of emotional intelligence and what areas might need some growth.

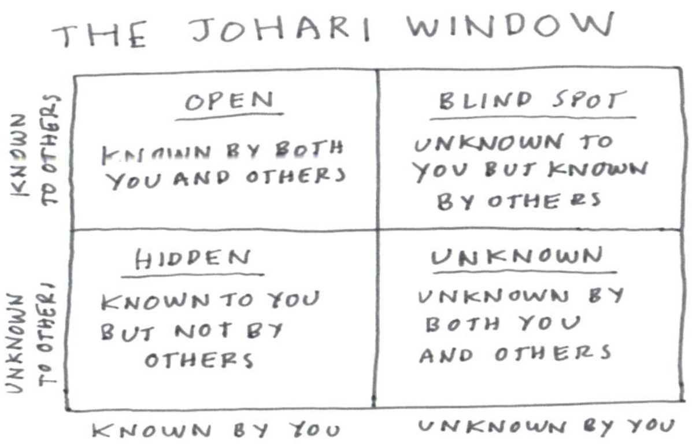

THE JOHARI WINDOW

	KNOWN BY YOU	UNKNOWN BY YOU
KNOWN TO OTHERS	OPEN KNOWN BY BOTH YOU AND OTHERS	BLIND SPOT UNKNOWN TO YOU BUT KNOWN BY OTHERS
UNKNOWN TO OTHERS	HIDDEN KNOWN TO YOU BUT NOT BY OTHERS	UNKNOWN UNKNOWN BY BOTH YOU AND OTHERS

TAKE THE QUIZ HERE:
https://kevan.org/johari

Send it to 5-7 people, friends, family, co-workers and then it will populate with the four quadrants. Providing you some insight on how YOU perceive yourself compared to how others perceive you.

Created by: JOSEPH LUFT AND HARRINGTON INGHAM

With this insight we can develop our emotional intelligence by expanding the "Open Area." As we increase the parts of ourselves that are known to self and to others, we enhance our ability to build effective relationships, both on and off the job, and especially when it matters most to you.

What was the most surprising difference between your response and that of those close to you?

____

____

SOCIAL AWARENESS

Social Awareness is the ability to observe and accept the perspective of, and empathize with, others from diverse backgrounds, cultures, and varying emotional reactivity. To also be aware of how we are perceived by others and appropriately modify our interactions with respect to the social and ethical norms for behavior in any given situation.

How we are perceived in our interactions has a lot to do with how well we gain our communication objectives. If we think of social awareness as interpersonal leadership, it will solidify the concept of how we influence interactional success. In his book, "***Leading from the Inside Out***", author Kevin Cashman said, *"We tend to view leadership as an external event . . . as something we do. Rather, leadership is an intimate expression of who we are; it is our being in action,"* a statement that can challenge our perception of leading as a "telling" position, so let's dissect some more. There is commanding when the situation requires absolute direction without question. Then there is leading, or influencing, which requires people to want to follow you. Adapting our manner of body language, words, tone, pitch, volume, and presence (or vibe), to get the best results to meet our interactive objective is utilizing high social awareness; reading others and environments to provide clues on how to present yourself and react accordingly. Difficult for those with spectrum disorders, narcissists, and some trauma injuries, so consider that when the behavior you are receiving seems bizarre and inappropriate for the moment. Situational awareness should take precedence for your safety and the safety of others.

BUILDING SOCIAL AWARENESS

1. Prepare to be mindfully present during an important interaction
2. Create a word or phrase that best represents the outcome you are looking for in that exchange
3. Step into the mood you wish to project (think of a happy, funny, thoughtful moment)
4. Make sure you are looking through a clear lens (challenge perceptions and bias)
5. Pay attention to the body language, pitch, volume, tone, and choice of words, yours, and theirs
6. Practice empathetic listening, clear your brain of responses and investigate the meaning of the words and body language you are listening to
7. Understand when ego states shift, and adapt the appropriate response for the outcome you have envisioned
8. Build curiosity and genuine interest in others in every possible interaction so this becomes second nature in all your strategic communications

Think of a situation where using this social awareness information would have benefited you with a better outcome? Which of the above tips would have been most useful?

____

____

____

When interviewing or seeking to gain information from others, becoming strategic in our verbal interaction becomes paramount.

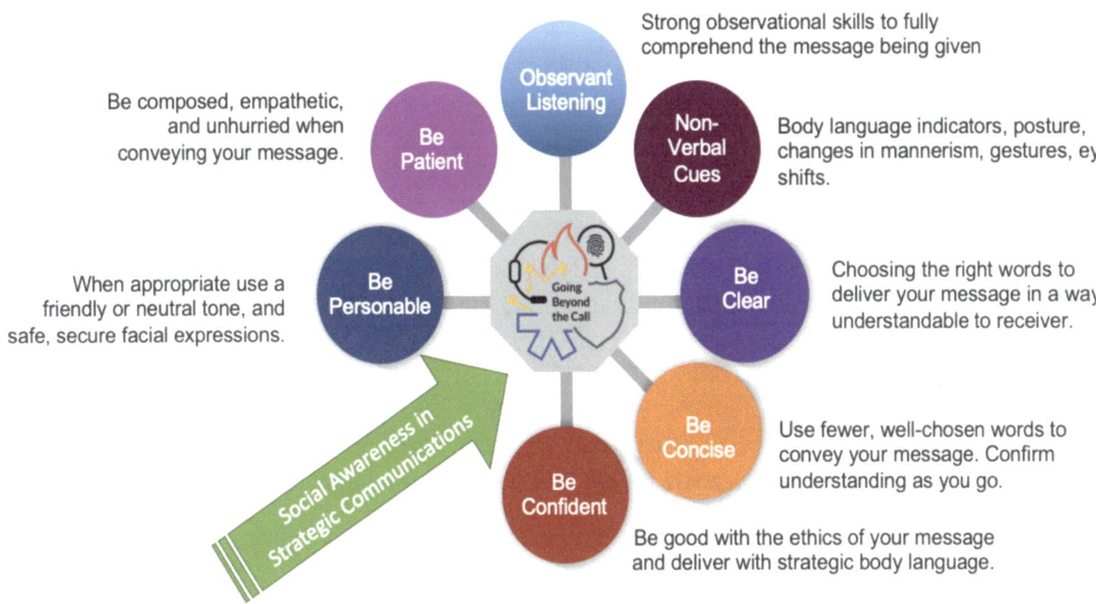

UNDERSTANDING EMPATHY

WATCH: Brené Brown on Empathy: https://youtu.be/1Evwgu369Jw

We share this video in our workshops as it summarizes empathy perfectly. Empathy allows us to become more socially aware and to better manage and influence our relationships. Self-Management is a prerequisite for healthy social awareness, and the effectiveness of how we read, interpret, and handle people. For our important relationships it helps with an awareness of another's feelings, needs, and concerns and build connective interactions. When we have better control over our self in this arena, we earn the right to build rapport in a manner where we can manage and influence interactions. Being socially aware also means that you understand how *you* react to different people and social situations which will help you effectively modify your interactive tactics with other people, so that you achieve the best results for all involved.

With empathy, we can understand or imagine the feelings and thoughts of others from their own perspective and have an active but distant role in their concerns. There is often confusion when we speak about empathy, and many confuse what they are actually feeling. Here is a comparison that makes it clearer.

PITY	SYMPATHY	EMPATHY	COMPASSION
I acknowledge your suffering	I care about your suffering	I feel your suffering	I want to relieve your suffering

Empathy increasing activity:

Choose 5 people you would like to improve your relationship with. Using the social awareness tips above have mindful conversations with each person.

I commit to the relationship builder exercise with the following five people:

1. ______________________________
2. ______________________________
3. ______________________________
4. ______________________________
5. ______________________________

Note the following: *Did I feel more empathetic and warmer (kind, respectful) to them? Did I gather more intelligence about what they said with this tactic?*

____

____

____

____

____

____

____

____

Did they react differently to me? What was different?
Did I achieve better communication outcomes using an empathetic approach?

____

____

____

____

____

____

____

No one cares how much you know, until they know how much you care.
-Theodore Roosevelt

SELF MANAGEMENT

"Integrity is telling myself the truth, and honesty is telling the truth to other people."
~ Spencer Johnson, author of Who Moved My Cheese.

1. Self-management or self-regulation refers to the act of taking responsibility for oneself, our emotions, and how they impact our decisions and behaviors. It is with strong integrity that we ask ourselves "do I control my emotions, or do my emotions control me?" Many will move through life with an "it is what it is" mindset rather than "it is what you make it" The later forces your personal responsibility towards awareness that we have control over how we manage what we face. Emotional Intelligent growth is very self-reflective. We have given you numerous insights to begin this journey throughout our program and this workbook.

2. Self-control – the ability to pause and think before acting. With trauma experiences it also means reflecting on one's negative choices, reframing bad psychological drivers, and building new skills and habits that better serve our desired state.

3. Trustworthiness – starts with trusting yourself, setting boundaries and building a set of core values that best reflect the person you want to be. It then expands to others by showing you will do as you say, say what you mean, and mean what you do rather than be controlled by maladaptive knee-jerk reactions.

4. Adaptability – means growing your resiliency, emotional controls, and toolbox to manage change from a thought mindset and not an emotional reactivity one. Change is the only constant and, in these professions, and normal course of duty. Add in the trauma events that will eat away at your core, if you do not manage it, and being flexible and comfortable with adapting to new norms is essential.

5. Achievement Orientation – understand whether you are motivated by avoiding pain or achieving gain and then plan, organize, and prioritize life goals utilizing your personal driver.

6. Initiative – in relation to self-management it is the willingness to act and get things done in your own best interest. When we refuse to settle for a low or burdened quality of life we are driven towards learning, growth, and improved mental fitness.

7. Accountability – assuming complete responsibility for your actions, and inactions. Deliver on your promises (including to yourself), admit mistakes, and avoid blaming.

Humans are motivated by the avoidance of pain or the achievement of gain.

Rate yourself on a scale of 1-10? This can be where you start to build an adaptive resiliency plan for advancing your self-management.

SELF MANAGEMENT	Scale 1-10										My Motivation	
Honest self-reflection	1	2	3	4	5	6	7	8	9	10	**PAIN**	**GAIN**
Self-Control												
Trustworthiness												
Adaptability												
Achievement Orientation												
Initiative												
Accountability												

What are you most surprised with? Jot down some ideas you have to improve lower areas of self-management.

____

____

____

BODY LANGUAGE

"If you had a hundred masks upon your face, your thoughts however slight would not be hidden from me." ~Dante Alighieri (Purgatorio, Canto XV)

Body language interpretation is the most misunderstood interaction tactic. So, while we share some general aspects of reading others, we do so with caution. Body language interpretation is a complex expertise to master and no one movement will give you absolute answers as a stand-alone tool. When used as cues to deepen, change, re-focus, or advance the continuation of your strategic communication, it can be a useful tool; but do not make conclusions on gestures and movements alone. As example, when anxious, apprehensive, disturbed, or simply bored, self-touch gestures can help us calm our nervous system. Using physical contact on oneself stimulates tactile nerve endings which will help refocus our stressor, moving inward and away from whatever is bothering our senses outside ourselves. Those who have underlying mental health challenges may do so as a fidget or habit versus any indication of guilt, lying, or misdirection. Also, those who witnessed something disturbing or are fearful or anxious of any aspect of the interaction may self-sooth.

Watching for baseline behaviors in others is the first step in understanding body language, and then use any changes to signal the moment to deepen the communication or adapt the interaction. Take the common belief that crossed arms or legs signals defensiveness; the reality is some people simply feel comfortable crossing their arms or legs, so it doesn't necessarily indicate defensiveness. However, when they shift away from that norm during key conversational points, THEN you have something to work with.

There are some universal facial expressions you should be familiar with and general body language interpretations that can be helpful in advancing your communication goals. Cultural norms, wanting to show off in front of others, and even some mental health disorders may alter what you perceive to be a normal expression or bodily reaction. Also remember, facial emotions and expressive body language does not tell you the underlying trigger; it could be a remembered feeling, experience, or trauma and unrelated to the conversation you are having. With this caution, please watch the following YouTube to have some fun decoding universal facial expressions. Dr. Paul Ekman (Ekman Group) has in-depth training on micro-expressions should you wish to pursue further expertise. We have a lot of fun with an interactive video exercise, "guess the expression" in our workshops. So have fun with it!

WATCH: Universal facial expressions: YouTube: https://youtu.be/B0ouAnmsO1Y

With others, knowing many hidden or buried triggers can influence how our face and body react to these emotional surges allows us more intelligence to peel the onion empathetically without assigning a conclusion prematurely. Building rapport with effective emotional intelligence and strategic communication allows one to obtain a good baseline and then consider the emotional spikes we observe from there.

Understanding basic micro expressions can be a wakeup call if you and your significant other are experiencing declining relationship health. From videotape studies of nearly 700 married couples in therapy sessions while discussing their emotional relationships with each other, University of Washington psychologist, John Gottman has found the sneer expression (even fleeting episodes of the cue) to be a "potent signal" for predicting the likelihood of future marital disintegration (Bates and Cleese 2001). In this regard, the sneer may be decoded as an unconscious sign of contempt. More on this in the next section.

Our faces can reveal a tremendous number of emotions, both conscious and often unconscious reactions reflect how we feel. When someone close to us fails to believe what we say due to the accompanying body language we often end up in arguments. Understanding ourselves, our moods, and self-observation on our body indicators can help build congruency between our conscious, subconscious, and both inward and outward facing communication.

Marc Brackett, Ph.D., Director of the ***Yale University's Center for Emotional Intelligence*** created the mood meter (below). He shares that we have a couple of thousand emotions running through our bodies every day on an average of 3-5 in a minute, think of it as a cascade of moving emotions. Many of us have difficulty identifying what emotion each moment brings us which can impact how effective we are at both self-talk and communicating with others. Like the emotion wheel we previously mentioned, Brackett's work helps us identify our moods and with that underlying and often hidden triggers. You can track your moods with apps or manually using the chart below and when you feel a mood, but not sure why, it can help you identify an area you may wish to dig a little deeper on. The mood tracking apps can help you with tracking your moods through the day and during different experiences if understanding your emotions is an area you wish to grow.

MOOD METER

High energy
Low pleasantness

High energy
High pleasantness

Enraged	Panicked	Stressed	Jittery	Shocked	Surprised	Upbeat	Festive	Exhilarated	Ecstatic
Livid	Furious	Frustrated	Tense	Stunned	Hyper	Cheerful	Motivated	Inspired	Elated
Fuming	Frightened	Angry	Nervous	Restless	Energized	Lively	Excited	Optimistic	Enthusiastic
Anxious	Apprehensive	Worried	Irritated	Annoyed	Pleased	Focused	Happy	Proud	Thrilled
Repulsed	Troubled	Concerned	Uneasy	Peeved	Pleasant	Joyful	Hopeful	Playful	Blissful
Disgusted	Glum	Disappointed	Down	Apathetic	At Ease	Easygoing	Content	Loving	Fulfilled
Pessimistic	Morose	Discouraged	Sad	Bored	Calm	Secure	Satisfied	Grateful	Touched
Alienated	Miserable	Lonely	Disheartened	Tired	Relaxed	Chill	Restful	Blessed	Balanced
Despondent	Depressed	Sullen	Exhausted	Fatigued	Mellow	Thoughtful	Peaceful	Comfortable	Carefree
Despairing	Hopeless	Desolate	Spent	Drained	Sleepy	Complacent	Tranquil	Cozy	Serene

Low energy
Low pleasantness

Low energy
High pleasantness

What is my most constant mood at work? At home? With friends? With loved ones?

____

____

____

RELATIONSHIP MANAGEMENT

Relationship Management reflects your interpersonal communication skills. Whether you want to inspire, influence, or get the best out of them in a situation how you approach and manage the communication garners the results. It is not about manipulation, domination, or control, it is about avoiding and resolving conflict and gaining the best possible objective in any communication. Without attempting to bond and find common ground the ability to manage and influence is lost.

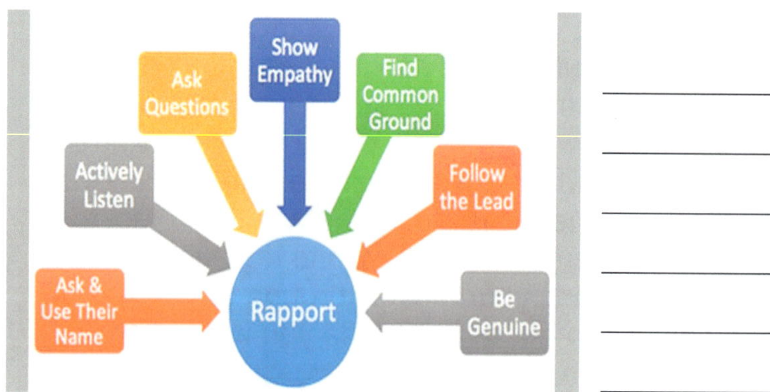

____

____

____

____

____

____

In your work and personal life your communication and relationship management skills need to be just as adaptive as your resiliency tactics. As you learn all the underlying elements that lead to interactive success you will find even the most difficult situations easier to manage. Different scenarios will require options for response and influence. By now we understand the command-and-control response is important when safety is a risk factor, but not always the best course of action to meet your interactive objective. At home, we can also default to a responsive norm that isn't always the most beneficial for our relationships. So, let's shift to the relationships that matter most as Going Beyond the Call is highly committed to helping your success off the job as well as when working. As with all other elements of mental fitness, this area also starts at birth and how we attach to others who are important to us. The attachment bond is the emotional connection you formed as an infant with your primary protective caregiver and is primarily associated to times of distress, illness, and tiredness. It is a critical developmental milestone that allows infants to learn to regulate their negative experiences and explore their known, new, or even more frightening environments.

WATCH: Attachment Theory: How Childhood Affects Life
https://youtu.be/WjOowWxOXCg

According to *attachment theory*, pioneered by British psychiatrist John Bowlby, and American psychologist Mary Ainsworth, the quality of the bonding you experienced during your initial relationship with your primary caregiver often determines how well you relate to other people and respond to intimacy throughout life. The Four Attachment Styles are: secure, anxious-preoccupied, dismissive-avoidant and fearful-avoidant. Understanding yours helps to course correct issues that were implanted long ago.

Choices	Attachment Descriptor	Your style	Your significant other's style
Secure	*Caregivers were sensitive to your needs and emotionally available. Responding appropriately to your early stressors. Adults with this style have generally healthy relationships, trust reasonably well, and it is fairly easy to get close and form connections. They are comfortable depending on others and do not fear abandonment.*		
Anxious-ambivalent	*This is an insecure attachment. Children are clingy and crave attention from their caregivers while they also may push them away. Adults tend to be jealous and not trust love or commitment from others. They have a strong fear of rejection, abandonment and dislike being alone. Adults will want to get very close and may scare off those close to them.*		
Anxious avoidant	*This is an insecure attachment. Children likely didn't feel comfortable seeking out their caregivers during distress. They may have been rejected and fended for themselves. Adults have a hard time trusting others and have a heightened sense of independence.*		
Disorganized Fearful avoidant	*This is an insecure attachment. Children can feel confused at times. The behaviors and actions of their caregivers were not consistent or abusive. Adults will seem nervous about getting close and take longer to establish intimacy. They may have swinging moods of emotional then aloof. This style is often seen in those with personality or mood disorders.*		

With your type identified, you will find it easier to identify patterns in your relationships. You may reflect on past romantic and friend relationships and discover where you may communicate and react in ways that sabotage your happiness and security. None of the options is considered good or bad, the aim is to provide more insight to consider when building resiliency and emotional growth for your self-awareness and relationship management.

WHY DO RELATIONSHIPS TYPICALLY FAIL?

1/ Unrealistic expectations
2/ Lack of empathy
3/ Low emotional intelligence
4/ Dependency / Co-dependency
5/ Inability to assert ones needs and wants
6/ Poor communication skills
7/ Ineffective strategies for conflict resolution
8/ Personality / Ego State emotionalized influence
9/ Different "love languages"
10/ Trauma influenced behavior changes
11/ Lack or loss of trust

YOUR OWN REASONS:

____

____

____

____

The most obvious indicator that a discussion is not going to go well between romantic partners is the way the conversation begins. When a discussion leads off with criticism and/or sarcasm, a form of contempt, it has begun with a harsh startup. John Gottman, author of What Predicts Divorce? reports, *"Statistics tell the story: 96 percent of the time you can predict the outcome of a conversation based on the first three minutes of the fifteen-minute interaction!"*

Gottman, who predicts divorce with over 90% accuracy, shares the most damaging communication styles calling them the Four Horsemen of the Relationship Apocalypse. They are Criticism, Defensiveness, Stonewalling, and Contempt.

WATCH: YouTube the Four Horsemen of the Relationship Apocalypse https://youtu.be/1o30Ps-_8is this video includes how to manage it. There are many resources on the Gottman site for turning around damaged relationships.

Due to the additional stress placed on public safety and other high stress careers, extra attention and care needs to take place to manage the best possible relationship. Shiftwork, high stress, sleep challenges, and trauma events battering away at your persona are only a few aspects that damage healthy relationships, and an emotionally intelligent partner will take the lead to mitigate the potential impacts.

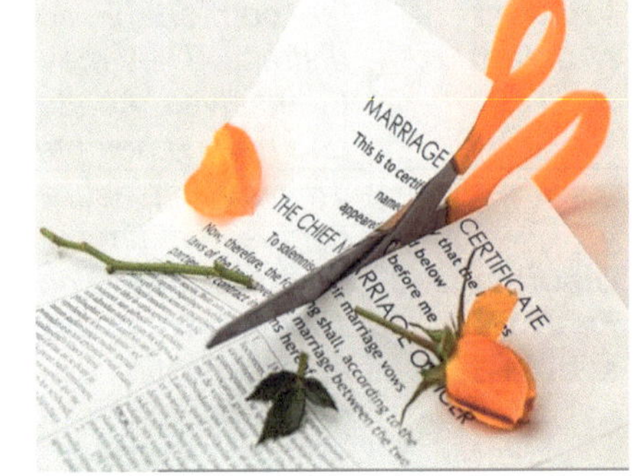

"While empathy is only one part of emotional intelligence, it can enable us to be less preoccupied with our well-being and more concerned with mutual well-being."
~ John Gottman

KNOW YOURS AND OTHERS LOVE LANGUAGE AND KEEP THEIR TANKS FULL!

GARY CHAPMAN'S 5 LOVE LANGUAGES – TAKE THE QUIZ https://5lovelanguages.com/quizzes/love-language	
Words of Affirmation	Verbal compliments that express your love, gratitude, and appreciation
Acts of Service	Any act that eases the others burden of responsibility
Quality Time	Focused and undivided attention spent together
Gifts	Tangible symbols that you are thinking of them and made effort to show it
Physical Touch	Nonsexual touch that reinforces how much you care. Intimate encounters that focus on their pleasure

	GOING BEYOND THE CALL - 5 LOVE LANGUAGES COMMUNICATION TACTICS		
	Actions?	**What to Avoid?**	**After Conflict?**
Words of Affirmation	• Share regular and specific reasons I like/ admire/respect/appreciate /love another. • Lots of compliments and affirmations. • Encouraging words, moments of pride. • Brag to others about them. • Write notes or send specific texts of good job /like /love/proud of...	• Emotionally harsh words. • Undue criticism. • Sarcasm • Jokes with them as the punching bag • Negative comments in front of others • Not verbally sandwiching bad with good. • Loud/overheard critique	• Initiate a sincere apology or make 1st steps towards peace for the conflict. • Speak in ways that rebuild security, trust, like or love • Confirm boundaries, if necessary, use positive reframing "I heard you..." • to commit to conflict issue resolution
Acts of Service	• Do chores/errands/duties without being asked. • Be helpful, take over efforts "let me do that for you", give w/o expectation of return. • Speak using "What can I do," "I will do this for you," Today, I did this for you."	• Forgetting promises. • Don't overcommit • Ignoring their stress with others, chores, duties. • Adding to their burden by creating more work. • Say "that's not my job" • Be derelict in your duty	• Initiate and change behaviors, actions, habits, or manners that caused conflict • Regularly ask "what can I do to make your life/job/duty/ easier type questions.
Quality Time	• Make anniversaries, birthdays extra special, turn off the TV, phone, and make one on one time, have a hobby or activity that just you two. • Undivided attention in one-on-one scenarios. • Lunch/walk meets	• Do not isolate or ignore them. • Make everything group plans • Avoid too long of a gap between one-on-one time. • Spend more time with others, electronics, hobbies over them.	• Make eye contact, • Active listening (no interruptions) w/ empathy. • Program tech to avoid interruptions. • Prioritize time together. • Initiate long hugs with significant other.
Gifts	• Remembering and making anniversaries and birthdays fun, wrap gifts with purpose/care, • Surprise them with small tokens or treats they would enjoy (doesn't have to be costly)	• Materialism without care (i.e., giving cash/gift cards), or obvious last minute drug store holiday or birthday gift shopping. • Forgetting a special event/anniversary • Employee recognition	A handwritten apology note. • With tech you can text a poem, funny meme, or songs with "I saw or heard this and thought you would like/love it" ...
Physical Touch	• Focused handshakes, fist bumps, shoulder/ elbow touches, back slaps. • Long hugs, caressing, extended kissing, massages, hand holding, frequent walk by touches. • Unselfish lovemaking	• Physical abuse or harsh/rough touch. • Corporal punishment. • Threats • Neglect • Solitary duties • Social isolation	• Longer handshake with sincere apology. • You ok shoulder/back hug/safe touch. • 4min. eye gaze, long hugs, comfort stroking, no words, breath matching, cuddling, hints of intimate touch

What is your love language? ___________________________________
How about those closest to you at home and work? Contemplate what behaviors and communication choices you can change to improve these relationships.

MANAGING INTERACTIONS

"People are fascinating. Be curious and genuinely interested in everyone you encounter, and you will be amazed at how interested they become in you." ~Harold Henderson, Mayor, Richmond Quebec

Are you better at finding problems or solutions? Either way, you're right!

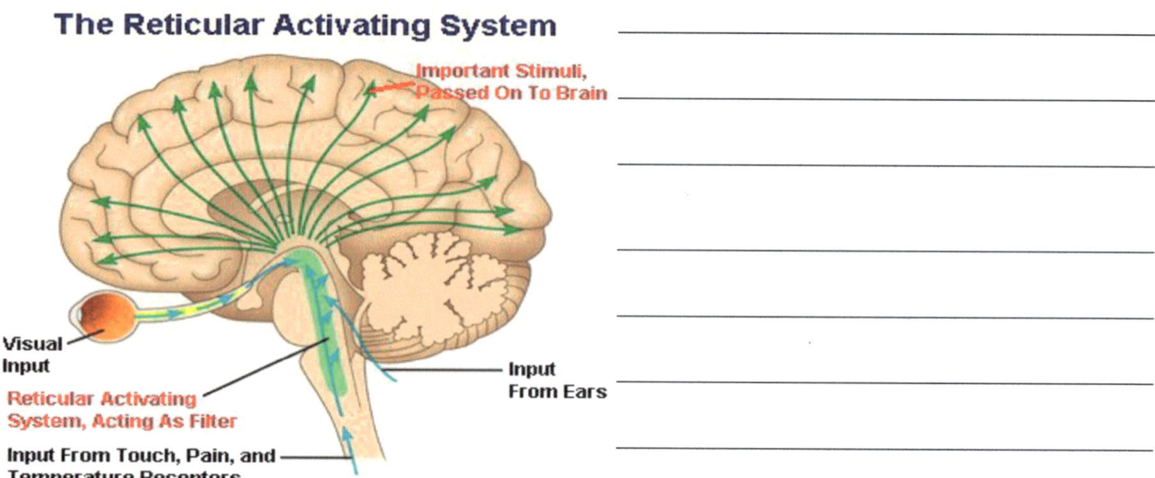

The Reticular Activating System (RAS) is nerve bundles in our brainstem, about the size of your finger. This network of neurons manages our sleep/wake cycle as well as takes in all input from your visceral, somatic, and sensory systems and then filters out unnecessary information so that the most important is passed along to your reactionary and cognitive functions. The RAS prioritizes threats (activating your fight, flight, freeze, and fawn response) before moving onto the new or novel, that which is deemed important to you (what you focus on), and finally the emotional impact or risk of the input. This is the reason you buy a new car and suddenly see it everywhere or can tune out a crowd but recognize your name being called.

Think of your RAS as a wonderous supercomputer in our brain that correlates everything against all knowledge, every experience, emotion, and physical impact, many we do not have any conscious recollection of. Based on the outcome of this process, it then decides what gets popped into the reactionary system (fight, flight, freeze, fawn), or up to our cognitive brain for considered thought. The RAS is the basis of self-fulfilling prophecies, as identified in the "Law of Attraction" (it seeks what we feed it as important) and may create habitual behaviors that do not serve us well. Since the brain can only process about 130 bits of data per second (in any meaningful way) this processing is critical, so that we do not become overwhelmed with the millions of incoming sensory inputs rendering us incapable of making decisions.

The good news is our RAS is programmable, we are what we give attention to. After threats, the RAS is seeking priority of that which is important to us and that which has particularly high emotional stamping. If our conscious brain is seeking negative, self-defeating, horrifying, inputs our brain will happily comply and seek out every possible aligned input to strengthen such thoughts.

Bias, self-damaging internal speak, and relationship failures can be improved by learning to re-program what we deem important. The following are some of the ways the RAS is not good for us when left to run amok without any controlled inputs and management.

RAS Bashing: Sometimes I surprise myself with negative thoughts about?

NEGATIVE THOUGHT	Feeling I get after (i.e., guilt, shame, disgust, confusion, etc.)	Reprogram RAS with new thought …
My self-talk		
A stereotype thought		
Judging without facts		
Only seeing the negative in a partner		

Part of managing negative thoughts is to actively develop positive thoughts which is easier when we have completed the self-work and know ourselves and our abilities well. We can then better assess our need for challenge to induce a flow state of happiness, at work and in our personal life. If we don't really understand ourselves, our value in life, or how to manage in influence those around us a victim state may set in. It may be difficult to build motivation towards aspirations, goals, and positive momentum. When we know ourselves well, we can explore our options to find the best possible happiness at work and home.

WATCH: FLOW https://youtu.be/8h6IMYRoCZw

"Many people assign certain power to concepts and things outside of themselves. Genuine human satisfaction arrives in a state of "flow." Where one feels alert, strong, in effortless control, unselfconscious, and achieving an optimal experience with the use of their uniqueness. Happiness is not a fixed state rather, it is developed with a focus on achieving flow in our lives, primarily through self-control. Achieved when we command the whirling mass of thoughts in our conscious and manage the inputs of the subconscious rather than letting those elements control us or letting other factors outside of ourselves rule when we have no control over them."

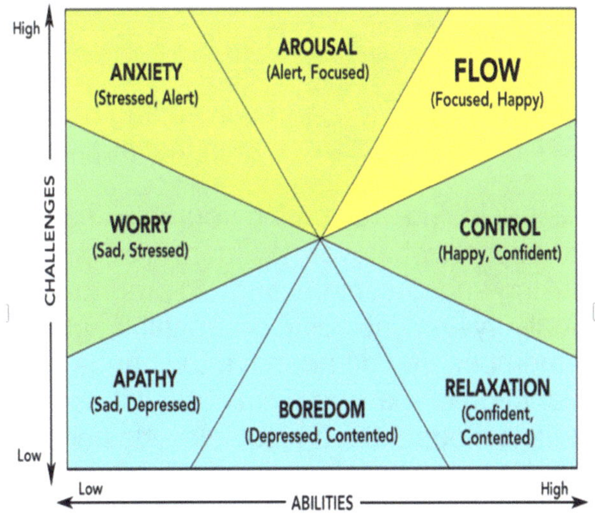

~ *Mihaly Csikszentmihalyi, (pronounced,* Cheek-sent-me-high)
Pioneer of the scientific study of happiness, author of Finding Flow

THE DARK SIDE - EMOTIONAL CONTAGION

Emotional Contagion as the spread of ideas, attitudes, or behavior patterns in a group through imitation and conformity, also known as behavioral contagion.

The RAS doesn't only influence our own internal thinking patterns, it has incredible impact on group dynamics. Manipulators, social media campaigns, marketing specialists, group organizers, politicians, all use this science to sway our opinion on what is important to us by manipulating our emotional responsiveness and heightening reactionary behavior. Maladaptive limbic systems impact people individually based on their experiences, but we like to be liked, we like being part of a tribe or group, and we like to hear like-minded group speak.

However, it is worth noting there is a dangerous side to this theory called social contagion which influences a group think mindset. Great at sporting events to get everyone riled up for their team however, it has a dark side. Whether in social circles, public events, within families, or even overarching as a group or organizational "culture", this may be an instigator. This can include:

Unconscious or conscious bias	Prejudice, unlawful actions	Rioting, mobs
People standing by and filming vs helping during a fight	Lack of decency behavior where people amass	Swarming

When has group think had you get caught up in something, that perhaps got out of hand?

____

____

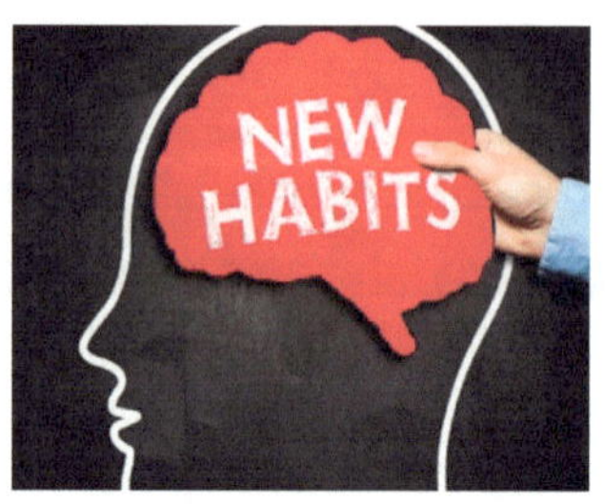

The good news is the brain has wonderous ability to change and adapt, so when we focus on automated inputs that do not serve us well and visualize and adopt new behaviors, we can change our RAS's filtering system to better benefit our goals and desires. In order to reprogram your RAS, you must change how your inputs are received and redirect your attention to new exposures, people, and things that support your intended outcomes.

This will include reshaping your thinking, biases, and core beliefs so that they better align and support whatever new norm you are working to cultivate. This means intentional thinking and deconstructing old programs that are looping and navigating your RAS's priority system including group think agendas that do not offer you a balanced perspective. Remember, you do not have to change your values, beliefs, or convictions to have a balanced perspective. Think about it as being a good debater, one that wants to be skilled and knowledgeable on multiple sides of an issue, so they are more intelligent and influential with their counter arguments.

What thought processes would I change first to improve my outlook towards myself, the world, and those in it?

____

____

RETICULAR ACTIVATING SYSTEM (RAS) CHANGE UP TIPS

1. Do a deep dive journaling exercise on automatic thoughts that do not serve you well.
2. Set goals for what you want to change, make them as visual and actionable as you can.
3. On a daily basis visualize a new way of thinking. This will reprogram the RAS where it begins to challenge automatic thoughts, notices new opportunity, is alerted that new evidence is being introduced. This will build coincidences, then momentum towards your goal(s).
4. Use the STOP, DROP, and ROLL technique to halt old automated, or goal defeating thoughts and give yourself grace when old programming seeps through. Like any program it can take some time to totally write over old data.

Stop automated thoughts that do not match the person you wish to project, or the inner dialogue you want to hear.

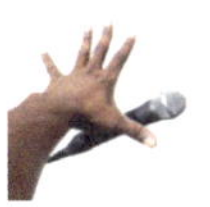

List what cognitive dissonance, bias, old, implanted thoughts from a social, environmental, family, cultural, or learned event. Drop the meaning programmed and write out a new meaning that aligns with the values you want moving forward.

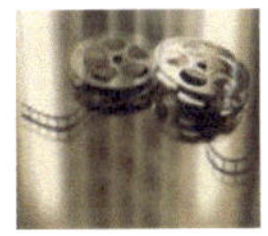

Roll out your new vision like a movie every day, be clear, definite, and creative in how this movie will play as your future programming takes hold.

This exercise may be challenging, especially the self-limiting inner dialogue. It may help to picture yourself giving the new RAS vision to someone you care for very deeply. Imagine being a family member, friend, or peer to someone you really wish you could get through to about their self-defeating talk. As you think of how to bolster their self-worth and self-imagine imagine you have great expertise in finding just the right words and suggested actions. Fill in the chart (or journal if room is required) and be as empathetic, caring, and specific as you can be.

VISION FOR NEW RAS PROGRAM	ACTION #1	ACTION #2

COMPLICATIONS IN COMMUNICATION
READ: CHAPTER 14

HUMOR CAN LIFT UP OR TEAR APART

Whether for general amusement of self or others or a coping mechanism humor is a great way to manage difficult feelings and change the state of the conversation. Whether that change is a positive or negative one is the question. There are four basic styles of humor discussed in psychological circles.

Affiliative humor is based on the enhancement of personal interactions with amusing remarks, joke telling, situational humor.

Self-enhancing humor is having a humorous take during adverse or harmful situations to Help ease self or others with emotional regulation.

Aggressive humor is consciously or habitually underscored with a sense of superiority Over others. It is subtly or overtly hostile and tends to hold element of truth even when purported to only be in jest.

Self-*defeating humor* is to seek social acceptance or the approval of others at one's own expense. Individuals who use this humor style tend to be avoiding managing internal conflict and hiding negative emotions.

Affiliative (situational), and self-enhancing humor styles are considered positive, adaptive humor, while aggressive and self-defeating humor are generally considered to have negative and damaging undertones. In these professions, a common coping mechanism is derogatory humor. When shared or with someone of alike humor styles, this can be a great stress reliever; however, when interacting with the public or at home it may well cause unnecessary conflict.

SARCASM	The use of irony to mock or convey contempt. It can be teasing, biting, or malicious
IRONY	The expression of one's meaning by using language that usually signifies the opposite, typically for humorous or emphatic effect
SATIRE	The use of humor, irony, exaggeration, or ridicule to expose and criticize people's stupidity or vices

How do you use humor? With your inner circle, does it enhance or damage relationships?

___

___

___

___

COMMUNICATION CHANNEL CAPACITY

WORDS ARE POWERFUL

People prioritize what they trust in the physiology, or the vibe they get off of you. A huge amount of interpretation rests on the verbal aspect so don't mistake the 7% as not being important, it is. The rest is just lie detection, as example, emphasize the bold word when saying this sentence, *"I never said she stole my money,"* and hear how many ways it can be interpreted:

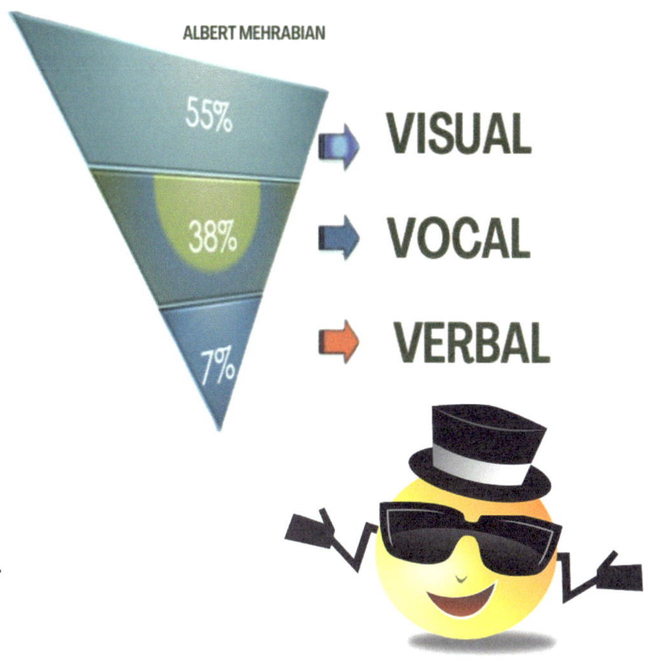

1. ***I*** never said she stole my money.
2. I ***never said*** she stole my money.
3. I never said ***she*** stole my money.
4. I never said she ***stole*** my money.
5. I never said she stole ***my*** money.
6. I never said she stole my ***money***.

BUT…I ***TOLD*** them…

How often do we stop to consider the manner in which we convey messages for optimum understanding? When has your message been completely misinterpreted by another? Think of how many times this happens in person, via video call, over the phone, or via text. Which ones were the worst misinterpretations?

___

___

___

___

___

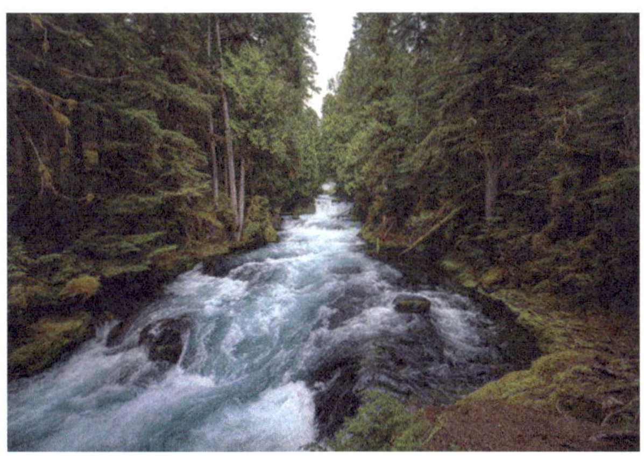

LANGUAGE IS LIMITED - READ RAGING RIVER in Chapter 14 (for answers)

We have a raging river of thoughts, feelings, experiences, biases, cultural influences, in every message we send, and we wonder why people don't "get us" or our message.

The more important the conversation or communication objective, the more critical our mode of communication becomes.

Think about this massive raging river of thoughts, memories, experiences, feelings, bias, cultural inputs, societal inputs, behind every important conversation you have, and all this background is experienced by seeing, hearing, and sensing your total meaning. Imagine a large raging river of all these internal meanings being pushed through these alternate flows:

Chapter 14 in GBTC book	*FILL IN THE BLANK*	*Answer*
FACE TO FACE IS LIKE A:		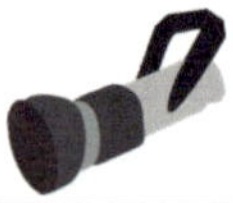
VIDEO CALL IS LIKE A:		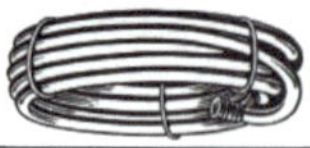
PHONE CALL IS LIKE A:		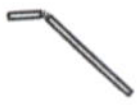
TEXTING IS LIKE A:		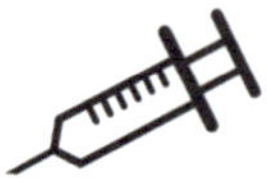

"Is the goal to TELL them or is the goal that they UNDERSTAND?"
~ James MacNeil

While the following also impacts your professional interactions, we want to focus this part of the workbook on personal growth. Anger and frustration are often misinterpreted and given your professions, there will be times your negative work experiences will come home with you and cause unnecessary challenges in your most valued relationships. The following is an exercise you can share with those close to you that can help all communicate from common understanding.

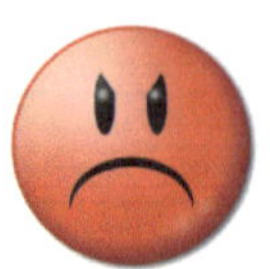

Hints of 'Anger' Exercise
(Homework assignment to use with family, peers, or friends)

Frustration, annoyance, and simply being in a bad mood are perfectly normal human emotions we all experience. For some, the body language, vibe, and communication style that comes with these emotions can often be confused with anger and cause unnecessary defensiveness or emotional escalation in another.

When confronted we may avoid, deny, or otherwise dismiss someone's interpretation that we are angry because that isn't how we feel, however, we haven't put cognitive thought in how we are presenting ourselves. Confusing emotional expression or interpretation can be especially true in our closest relationships, where, as example, we may want to protect a significant other from a disturbing or distressing situation that is weighing on our minds. Controlling how we present ourselves and ensuring others are receiving the message we wish to project will enhance your quality of life.

This activity will help you and others identify anger escalating cues in the pre-escalation stage before minor negative feelings develop into interaction or communication outcomes that unnecessarily intensified and often, later regretted. Tell the participating family/peer members to think about a time when they were quite angry or upset, and really identify how they felt mentally and physically.

Using the emotion wheel or mood meter from earlier in the workbook, each of you answer the following questions about how you felt when very angry?

1. **What were my moods throughout the conflict?**
2. **What kind of thoughts was going through your head?**
3. **Were your muscles relaxed or tight with tension?**
4. **Were your hands relaxed or clenched in a fist?**
5. **Was your heart rate normal or beating fast?**
6. **Did you have any cognitive distortions, self-defeating beliefs, other emotion expanding experiences?**

____

____

____

____

____

____

____

____

____

____

Moving forward use the emotion wheel, or mood meter app and do this exercise when you feel frustrated, annoyed, perturbed, disgusted, and other negative emotions that have been regularly misinterpreted by those close to you. Together, review your answers and discuss the discrepancies between what you think about your emotional cues and what other family members think and vice versa. You can come up with agreed upon statements or body language alterations that diffuse or alter escalation in the future. As example, when frustrated you may clench your fists, cross your arms, raise your voice trying to hold in what is bothering you. In the future you can agree to relax your body language and state, *"I'm not angry, just annoyed about a situation at work that is bothering me, but it isn't something I feel is appropriate to bring home, so give me some time to unwind. Sorry if my mood is dampening family time."*

INFLUENCING OTHERS ETHICALLY **Read: Chapter 17 and 18**

"It is much more agreeable to offend and later ask forgiveness than to be offended and grant forgiveness. The one who does the former demonstrates his power and then his goodness. The other, if he does not want to be thought inhuman, must forgive; because of this coercion, pleasure in the other's humiliation is slight."
~ Friedrich Nietzsche, Aphorisms on Love and Hate

While self-awareness and management are the starting grounds, much of advanced emotional intelligence comes down to social awareness. It focuses on the ability to read other people, to be curious about their motivations and drivers and to consider what they are going through at the moment. Over time, this skill makes you an exceptional judge of character. You develop an understanding of their underlying influencers and motivations. You become difficult to offend as you build a firm understanding of who you are with strong self-control and other-person awareness. Others' opinions and viewpoints do not trigger you, which creates more open-mindedness along with incredible adaptive resilience both in communication and stress management. With self-control comes a stronger ability to manage and influence others.

The greatest tactic you can develop in social awareness is to hone your intuition, meaning your ability to read your own emotions and to understand how you are affected by others, and read others as they are influenced by inputs around them, including you. It is a fundamental survival skill. The open-loop limbic system describes the way others affect us. Our emotions are developed and projected based on the dynamics of several structures that make up our limbic system. Some internal systems are either closed loops, like our circulatory system, or sequential, like our digestive system. Our limbic system is considered an open loop by neuroscientists, and it is strongly adaptive and responsive to stimulus outside the body.

Think about a time someone walked into a room and immediately changed the vibe of all present, with a positive or negative vibe for all, or perhaps just your emotional state. Describe that experience:

____

____

When you walk into a room, do you usually lift up the vibe or dampen it?

____

EMOTIONAL CONTAGION

Our emotions can be altered by a person or a groups' emotional influence. An excellent example of this is any championship sporting event where the crowds create a vibe of excitement and competitiveness. Another example would be a rally, where groupthink can ignite and maintain united chanting, even turning ugly when protesters lose all sense of decency and decorum. We can also recognize this when someone walks into a room with a certain presence or attitude that impacts your state. Your conscious mind will pick up the change in milliseconds, calculating what change in the environment occurred and inputs a reaction to it based on your emotional history.

When that infecting person enters the room, shifting the vibe and instigating the change, we tend to point to them as the issue. However, the fact is you did not read *their* emotions, you read your emotional response to them. Managing this interactive experience gives you great influence, and we want you to manage that ethically.

If you want to present yourself powerfully, ensure you are congruent in your words, body language, and vocal aspects and you must be ethical in your approach. We all know the feeling of our hairs raising up because something is “off” about someone. Fake will be found out, even if it takes a while to come to that conclusion, your brain is on guard when presented with incongruence. Ethical congruence is especially important when your objective is to improve relationships or build quick rapport. You want to say what you mean and mean what you say. You must genuinely be curious, open, safe, and intent on the best possible outcome for all involved.

The cornerstone of being an effective communicator is to project a calm, safe, confident presence in order to achieve the best interactive objective. People are attracted to and comforted by a calm demeanor; more so when the situation is influenced by an emotionalized or traumatic moment. This cornerstone is equally important professionally and with our most valued personal relationships.

Think of the most trustworthy person you know. What about them conveys ethical influence in their body language, words, tone, pitch, volume, and vibe (or presence)?

____

____

____

Powerful strength comes from projecting a safe confidence, but not an egocentric confidence, an important difference. A powerful presence rarely brags; however, you instinctively know they are heroic. When they walk into the room, everyone notices, and they will often be described as a person with humility. It has been said that humility is not thinking *less of myself* it is merely ***thinking about myself, less***. That is the vision we wish to share for having calm, safe confidence, and a pure, ethical presence.

That does not mean denying yourself moments of war storytelling or sharing a heroic act. Not only does it help your brain deliver those memories to a safe long-term memory center but also, the world needs to hear about those accomplishments, and we all need a healthy amount of attention. Understanding our needs when it comes to how we feel valued, can significantly improve all our important relationships.

How does it work? Understanding that our brains can only process so much, so the subconscious has greater influence than we know. Based on what you have learned so far, you now know that as a recipient. Now we need to share how to project, manage, and influence others to gain the best possible outcome for all.

SELF-MASTERY -Read Chapter 12

"If we buy into the varying values of humanity, we will seek to impress those above, control those below and use or ignore the rest."
~ James MacNeil, Verbal Aikido

There is a commonality among all religions and spiritual practitioners, known as the golden rule. There is a slight wording variation, but the core message is, ***"do unto others as you would have others do unto you."*** If we humans followed no other interactive law than this one, the world would be a much kinder place. We do not though, so self-mastery involves determining what our internal self is meant to be and how we wish to project it to the world around us.

Basic human values are most often considered inherent values across humanity. The most common are honesty, loyalty, truth, love, peace, justice, good behavior, spiritual freedom, and self-management in conforming to the cultural and societal norms of our regional environment. We expect fundamental goodness in most humans and are disappointed when this isn't the case, which, in these professions, can happen at a higher percentage than the average human experiences. Therefore, self-mastery will require a more adaptive resilience to the harshness you encounter on a regular basis lest you become embittered to the human experience as it is supposed to be experienced. Those who experience repeated psychological trauma can also face this challenge from a defeatist mindset, sinking into mental health disorders, numbing, or detaching from the emotional experience of being human. When you have two groups coming together from opposing perspectives, experiencing similar psychological trauma at an above average rate, it is no wonder we have discord and conflict.

List your human values in order of importance to you, if there is one missing that is valuable to you then add it in. For inspiration check out Berne Browns list here: https://brenebrown.com/resources/dare-to-lead-list-of-values/

1. ______________________________
2. ______________________________
3. ______________________________
4. ______________________________
5. ______________________________
6. ______________________________
7. ______________________________
8. ______________________________
9. ______________________________
10. ______________________________

The secret of Pure Presence is being ... Fully Engaged and Fully Detached
~James MacNeil, Verbal Aikido

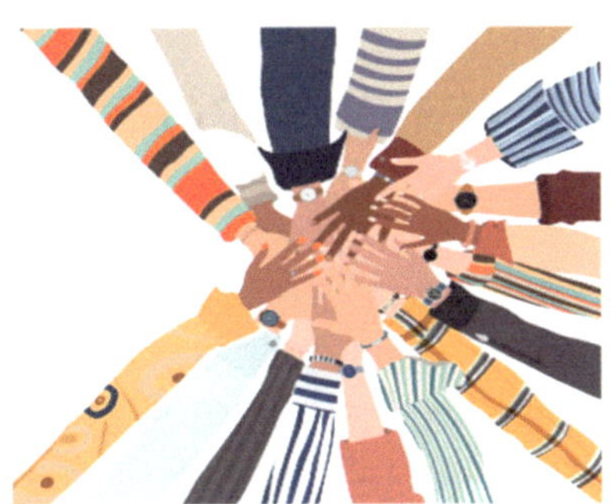

Human Values provide our basic attitudes, motivation, accepted behaviors, and rules of considerate co-existence. They influence our perception of the world, and our understanding of right and wrong. It impacts how we view our human organization, or 'pecking order' of those within our tribe circles; as well as place value on those who live outside our direct circles but still hold influence over us from a political, social, and economic perspective.

With the internet we are more exposed to the variations of accepted and common human practices, and it can add to the general distress we put on our psyche if we do not develop our ability to remain fully engaged, while completely detached. In all this people management, we want some level of control, and the shrinking world of modern society gives us less and less control as we march into the future.

The gift of acceptance even when someone's values are different than ours is priceless. It can be an enlightening experience to truly understand another's perspective and drivers without judgement. Even within family units this can be helpful to understand why we are unable to persuade someone or "get" their thinking. It can also be challenging when another's values differ from our cultural, spiritual, and political ones. This exercise teaches us to detach from our emotional selves and accept or be empathetic to something foreign to our thinking.

Rate these values on a scale of 1-10. Add to this list to fully incorporate values important to you. Now have the person you are closest to prioritize as well, or your kids, family, and friends. Be curious and non-judgmental about any valuations are different. Learn different perspectives and grow your emotional intelligence to comprehend we can be different variations of the same basic humanity. Be fully engaged, but fully detached from the outcome.

Your Common Human Values	1	2	3	4	5	6	7	8	9	10	*Your Significant Others' Human Values*
Honesty											*Honesty*
Loyalty											*Loyalty*
Truth											*Truth*
Love											*Love*
Peace											*Peace*
Justice											*Justice*
Good behavior											*Good behavior*
Spiritual freedom											*Spiritual freedom*
Self-management											*Self-management*

POWER OF PERCEPTION

For situations where cooperation is the primary objective and safety is not an immediate factor, the onus on the authority figure is to take command and control without presenting so much authority that you prevent a bond of trust to be established. Pre-escalation is the ability to find common ground, build rapport, gain co-operation, and ensure the best possible outcome given the circumstances being managed. By understanding some of the psychological and human behavior factors that lead to escalated interactions, you have more resources to find a starting point you can both agree upon. You also have a better chance at building fast rapport to move the moment from an "us-versus-them" situation to an "us" managing a situation together towards the best possible outcome.

There are three aspects to rapport: trust, likeability, and resonance. Ideally, we have all for ultimate rapport, the place where great relationships thrive. Of course, not all interactions are meant to build into relationships. In the book *The Speed of Trust: The One Thing that Changes Everything*, author Stephen M.R. Covey explains there are some people we like, but we don't trust. There are some people we trust, but we don't like. We can love someone's 'vibe' at an event, as example, but not really like them as a person or trust them in a more personal relationship. When working to build an interactive rapport with someone, trust is the place to start, especially when the situation or environment is tense.

Covey states: "*There is one thing that is common to every individual, relationship, team, family, organization, nation, economy, and civilization throughout the world—one thing which, if removed, will destroy the most powerful government, the most successful business, the most thriving economy, the most influential leadership, the greatest friendship, the strongest character, the deepest love. On the other hand, if developed and leveraged, that one thing has the potential to create unparalleled success and prosperity in every dimension of life. Yet, it is the least understood, most neglected, and most underestimated possibility of our time. That one thing is trust.*"

Fill in the blanks for understanding the difference between trust, liking, and resonance.

PERSON	LIKE	TRUST	HAS GREAT VIBE
E.G. The Boss, she is fair with assignments, relaxed, great storyteller, funny, and has our back but she is an attention seeker and flirt so I wouldn't like her in my inner circle.	✗	✓	✓

Building rapport through common ground and trust becomes an important skill to successfully maintain peaceful encounters. This is best accomplished when common ground is desired on both sides and with purposeful focus on a common objective. This is not an easily achieved. Most of the people you interact with will likely be in crisis, and the responsibility to create space for a respectful approach and engagement will fall squarely on your shoulders.

Demonstrating respect regardless of differences is an area where public safety professionals should have an advantage. As a paramilitary organizational structure, you are more aware of respect and acquiescence when it comes to hierarchy, even when you disagree with an order, policy, or practice. You understand the concept of respecting 'the thing' without agreeing with the person or policy behind it. The idea of respecting others whose behavior or actions fall outside of your preference is certainly more challenging; however, since the underlying goal is to avoid escalation, this initial rapport building tactic of showing respect works to your advantage.

To be clear, we are not advocating belief in or agreement with another's choice of actions when we use the word respect. We are advocating for respect for the human dynamic to achieve the objective of a safe and effective outcome in the situation you are managing. We are promoting understanding that the human condition is much more fragile and wrought with trauma than we usually consider. We are saying that your power position is stronger when you can empathize and first treat that human with the respect of meeting them where they are at and leading them to the best possible outcome for all. Finding common ground and building rapport gives you a powerful advantage in preventing escalation.

"If we had to agree on everything before communicating well with someone, we would never get anything accomplished," observes Deirdre von Krauskopf.

Often our bias and perception hinder our ability to present a respectful demeanor. When we can alter our perspective in an instant to gain the presence we wish to present, we gain significant people management and influence. Learning to change our paradigms at can change every interaction you have from here on out.

CHANGING PERSPECTIVE IN AN INSTANT: WATCH: Stephen Covey, 7 Habits of Effective People a video on changing Paradigms: https://youtu.be/w5XpMg53K4c

How did this story impact how you can alter how you see a situation? Think of a situation where your perception, or paradigm, about someone changed with new information.

Change the perception, and the experience changes. Consider that your original thought or belief was made up.

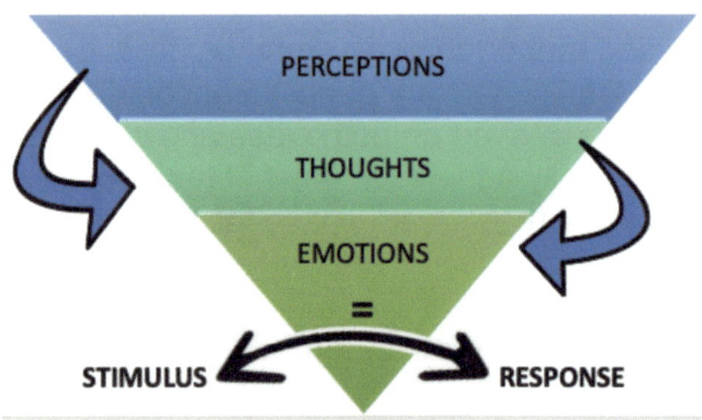

It was based on your past experiences, feelings, biases, culture, and assessed by the external inputs of the moment. The person next to you could have had a completely different reaction based on their processing of the same data.

Self-Management means controlling your response, not reacting blindly to the stimulus!

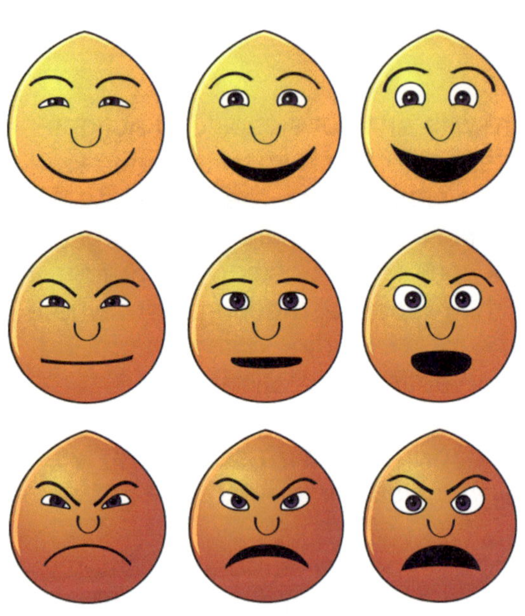

CHANGING STATE EXERCISE

Take a negative experience or memory (not too traumatic but one that eats at you a little). Find a relaxed location where you feel safe and will remain uninterrupted for a while. The goal is to neutralize the impact of that negative experience with changing or adapting your thinking about it.

Neutrally observe the experience, how it happened, where it was, who was there, how you felt about it, how you reacted initially and ongoing, and how you felt about it. Now analyze your feelings about it. ***What is it about each segment that bothers you or riles you up? When did you first feel this way about similar situations? How has this belief or way of thinking helped you or hindered you? Does this way of remembering have any value today?***

Now have some fun with it and change the various perceptions, biases, and beliefs about what you perceived others to be thinking or doing. If you change your belief system about the experience completely, how different does it look? What if your emotional intelligence was different and your self-beliefs were different? What if your emotions were not as intense, you had no concern about the outcome or financial aspect?

To change your perception is not about denying the event as it was initially experienced. It is merely changing your internal inputs and processing to view it from a different vantage point, or through different eyes. By attaching a different meaning, you can remove some of the emotional attachment and logically assess implications that will serve you better.

In your journal document the experience and your feelings towards altering the emotional impact of a negative event to control your emotional triggers.

COMMUNICATIONS SCIENCE PROFILE **Read: Chapter 19**

GoingBeyondTheCall.com | info@goingbeyondthecall.com

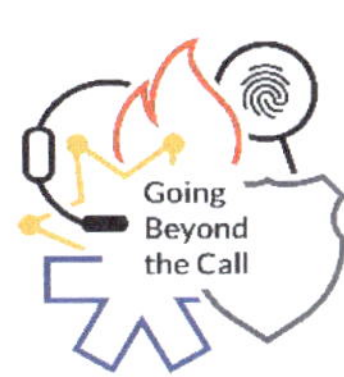

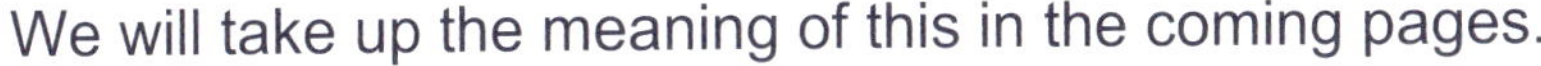

We will take up the meaning of this in the coming pages.

Indicate to what extent each description reflects you ***from the perspective of what others say***

1 =According to others, not true of me at all; 10=According to others, completely true of me

Circle the number that represents you the best. Go with your first thought as much as possible

Some people have said I am strong-minded. I easily see what is not right, and express what needs to be corrected or is not perfect. I live by rules and am disciplined. I act out my strong values where I can.

1 2 3 4 5 6 7 8 9 10

Some people have said I am helpful. I easily see where support is needed, and offer comfort where I can, or protect where there's a need. I give and I forgive. I am sympathetic, warm, and kind so as to encourage others.

1 2 3 4 5 6 7 8 9 10

Some people have said I am responsible. I easily see what is illogical because I am analytical. I gather all the information I can and express my thoughts rationally. I am present in the moment and act respectfully. I think things through and show consideration.

1 2 3 4 5 6 7 8 9 10

Some people have said I am carefree. I easily feel optimistic and happy and can be charmingly persuasive. I am curious, inventive, competitive, and/or playful. I live actively and enjoy showing affection. I can act on impulse.

1 2 3 4 5 6 7 8 9 10

Some people have said I am sensitive. I easily feel defensive and apologize. I reflect a lot and can be tearful. I enjoy spending time alone and I am comfortable being quiet. I feel overwhelmed and disengage.

1 2 3 4 5 6 7 8 9 10

Some people have said I am reactive. I easily see when things are placed in my way and say when these make me annoyed or frustrated. I believe I have to defend and protect myself when needed. I use strong language to show the intensity of what I feel.

1 2 3 4 5 6 7 8 9 10

Some people have said I am self-assured. I easily see my own goodness and know where I'm going with myself. I live by setting meaningful objectives, and work to achieve them. I am the kind of person I want to be.

1 2 3 4 5 6 7 8 9 10

TRANSACTIONAL and STRUCTURAL ANALYSIS - BEYOND PERSONALITY

Dr. Eric Berne, a Canadian, and US Military psychologist, developed transactional analysis and it is often used by therapists. When Deirdre studied Dr. Berne, she found his work to be a fantastic way to tie triggered trauma responses and the impact of social/emotional interactions to behavior and communication responses. It helps us understand how emotionalized reactivity overrides our perceived base personalities and how we can better manage our interactions, and influence others behavioral responses. We all have identifiable personalities we are born with that are influenced by the nature and nurture perspective. Our underlying Ego States are what we want to understand for strategic communication. How we act and react when emotionalized can be quite different from our day to day "personality." Berne defined an Ego State as *"a consistent pattern of feeling and experience directly related to a corresponding consistent pattern of behavior."*

Transactional Analysis (TA) is based on the notion that there are three sides, our 'Ego States' that emotionally drive our personalities, Parent, Adult and Child, that work together in internal and external communication in what Dr. Berne coined as transactions. Transactional Analysis data indicates that we tend to be dominated to varying degrees, based on the situation and people associated, by one of these three sides in emotional reactivity. Dr. Berne (1950) purported human relationships are a "repetitive sets of social maneuvers that serve a defensive function and yield important gratifications." Such maneuvers take the form of "games" that people play. These are relationship communication cycles, but they can also be more elaborate and follow an unconscious life plan or "script." Self-study and counselling TA can provide insights to our behavior and responsiveness, the games these lead to, and the scripts we live by when in certain situations. TA is a helpful tool for our own self-knowledge and personal development as well as a strategic communication tactic to manage and influence conversations and understand relationship dynamics.

Consider a large and repeated social or family event, a holiday ritual perhaps. Are there times when the same two, or more, people have the same argument every time? Are there personalities that seem to emotionally explode around certain people or topics discussed and instigators that poke that personality every time? Write out one of these scenarios to follow as we go through this section.

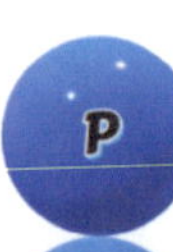	**Behaviors, feelings, and thoughts mimicked from parents or parental figures, split into two, our critical parent side and our nurturing parent side.**
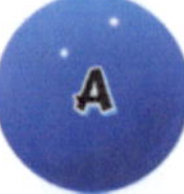	**Behaviors, feelings, and thoughts that directly respond to the here and now.**
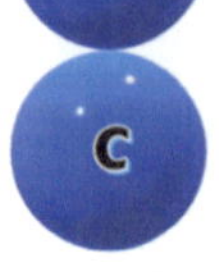	**Behaviors, feelings, and thoughts that are subconsciously replayed from our earliest childhood emotional responsiveness. Three aspects of natural child states are withdrawn, spontaneous, and angry.**

EGO STATE IDENTIFIERS

NATURE + NURTURE + EGO STATE DEVELEOPMENT = EMOTIONALIZED COMMUNICATION

Circle the characteristics in each that most suit you. You will see yourself in each and more in some. One tends to dominate in emotionalized, stressful, or triggered events. We may tend to choose what we wish we were like (self-projection) versus our true natural responsiveness.

Having a few close family and friends complete a profile on us as well can help bring fair and reasonable averages to your investigative and development potential. Does this analysis match the Communications Science Profile you and others completed?

PARENT EGO STATES		ADULT	CHILD EGO STATE (COUNTER TO THE ADULT)	FREE CHILD EGO STATE Broken down by type for easier identification			ADAPTED CHILD EGO STATE
CRITICAL PARENT	NUTURING PARENT		LITTLE PROFESSOR	SPONTANEOUS	WITHDRAWN	ANGRY	TRAUMA/ABUSE
Morals	Encourages	Responsible	Manipulative	Playful	Cautious	Brave	World is not OK
Values	Helpfulness	Thoughtfulness	Intuitive	Goofy	Selfish	Reactive	Avoids confrontation
Teaches	Protectiveness	Respectful	Curious	Laughter	Deep thinker	Frustration	Fear of punishment
Disciplines	Supportive	Considerate	Persuasive	Teasing	Introverted	Temper	Adapts to Should, Ought, Musts
Decisiveness	Giving	Reasonable	Charming	Optimistic	Shy	Defensive	Dysfunction is norm
Judgements	Forgiving	Analytical	Creative	Affectionate	Whiny	Demanding	Rely on survival skills
Standards	Comforting	Rational	Fantasy	Humor	Sensitive	Argues	Brought up on don't be, do, act
Set Rules	Sympathizing	In the present	Inventive	Competitive	Peacefulness	Lashes out	Unheard
Corrects/Fixes	Empathizes	Assertive	Believe in magic	Active	Easily startled	Brazen	Feelings are valued
Punishes	Guides	Logical	Calculating	Uncontrolled	Disengages	Threatening	Do what I say, not what I do modeling
Restricts	Coaches	Self-care	Self-promoting	Lacks caution	Apologetic	Selfish	Hypervigilant
Mentors	Warmth	Ideas driven	Assertive	Jumps all in	Quiet	Immature	Any attention is good attention, even evil
Instructs	Kindness	Considers new input	Driven	Silly	Defensive	Aggressive	Lacks trust in self and others
Creates Boundaries	Caring	Weighs pros & cons	Helps others	Nuisance	Tearful	Win at all costs	Unresponsive / Acts out against authority

We all manifest the three in different degrees and responsiveness to varying stimuli. You may act very different when annoyed at work than when annoyed by a sibling at a family event. Your basic personality is influenced by these emotionalized aspects. It is why drastically different emotional responsiveness can happen among siblings. Or when that person you work with has an emotional blowout that seems very uncharacteristic to them. What happened to lead to that response? What was the personality traits and ego state communication choices that preluded the response? The more we observe and practice this science, the better strategic communicators we become.

CHILD STATE: A regressive auto response of the individual's archaic past, our, "archaeopsyche" developed from birth to the time external norms and environment influenced behavior. There is a natural child state and an adapted child state if trauma, abuse, or extreme situational or environmental stress enters the early development stage.

PARENT STATE: The next stage of development comes from the parents, guardians, and key adults that imprint on us from birth to when we start taking in more outside influence from other people, TV or media, and environments (like school). Identified as our "Exteropsyche."

ADULT STATE: The third stage arrives when we start to form an independent view of how we see and react in the world (think about the terrible twos in infant development) where we challenge the expected influence of the primary adults in our world and work to form our own reactivity to stimuli and communication. As we grow and mature this becomes our logic, reasoning, and "data-processing" part of self, or the "neopsyche."

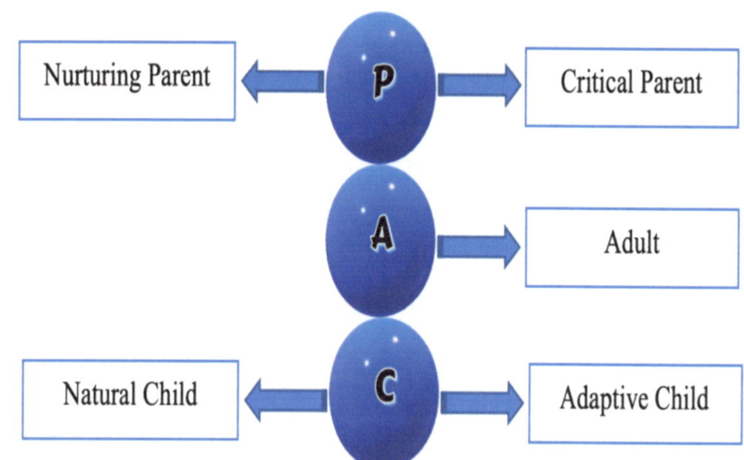

Each of these emotionalized aspects of the person perceives reality differently: the child part is perceived pre-logically and distortedly; the parent part, judgmentally and how we care about others; and the adult part, how we comprehend and consider on the basis of past experience.

What is the most interesting finding about this science? How do you think it will help your more vital relationship conversations?

____

____

____

Now go back and look at your results from the Communication Science Profile. If you haven't done this already, this is a great exercise to share with 5 – 10 close family and friends to see how others perceive you. Journal any differences and reflect on how different people influence your emotional reactivity in difference environments. When we understand ourselves in this way, it becomes easier to identify and assess others. With this skill we can adapt our communication approach to influence the conversational outcomes we are striving for.

MY PERSONAL ASSESSMENT OF MYSELF: ______________________________

DIFFERENT ASSESSSMENTS BY:

THE PERSON YOU ASKED TO RATE YOU | **THE PRIMARY EGO STATE THEY IDENTIFIED**

PERSON: ____________________ PRIMARY EGO STATE: ____________________

PERSON: ____________________ PRIMARY EGO STATE: ____________________

PERSON: ____________________ PRIMARY EGO STATE: ____________________

You can also compare your scores to the North American averages (on the next page), and where psychology experts indicate the optimum value is. There is no right or wrong overall, simply an awareness of where you are, how you react, and if there is room for growth if your current reactions are not getting you the results you want.

Think about your significant other, children, siblings, cousins, or really close friends and based on what you have learned so far, which of these Ego States do they seem to default to when they are upset about something?

PERSON: ____________________ DEFAULT EGO STATE: ____________________

PERSON: ____________________ DEFAULT EGO STATE: ____________________

PERSON: ____________________ DEFAULT EGO STATE: ____________________

EGO STATES: TOO MUCH ~ JUST RIGHT ~ TOO LITTLE

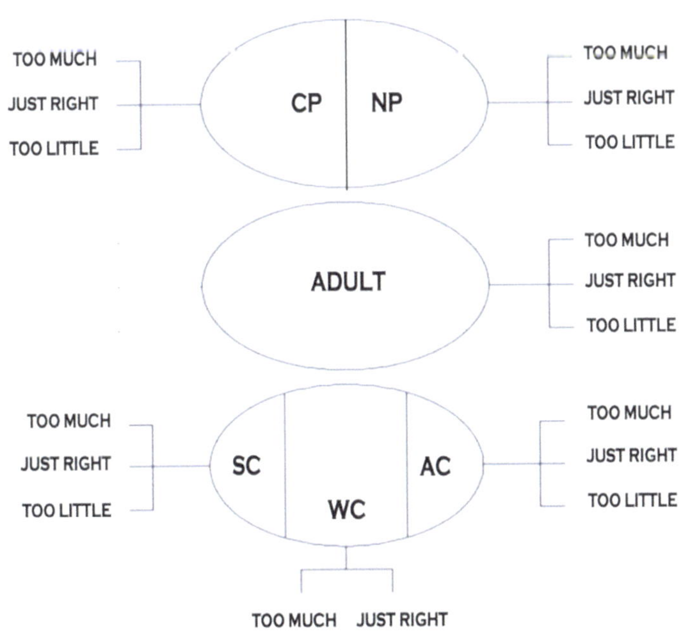

Where personal development comes into play is where we find that one or more of our Ego States is too much or too little.

We also want to investigate our closest relationships and see where our approach may not be getting the best communicative responses. Moving into Structural Analysis allows us to understand we tend to receive a response based on what we project.

Circle any areas you feel you may be too much or too little.

Communication Science Profile

Indicate to what extent each description reflects you from the perspective of what others say

1 – According to others, not true of me at all
10 – According to others, completely true of me

Circle the number that represents you the best. Go with your first thought as much as possible

Some people have said I am strongly-minded. I easily see what is not right, and express what needs to be corrected or is not perfect. I live by rules and am disciplined. I act out my strong values where I can. **Critical Parent**

1 . 2 . 3 . 4 . 5 . 6 . 7 . 8 . 9 . 10 ___ **CP**

Some people have said I am helpful. I easily see where support is needed, and offer comfort where I can, or protect where there's a need. I give and I forgive. I am sympathetic, warm and kind so as to encourage others. **Nurturing Parent**

1 . 2 . 3 . 4 . 5 . 6 . 7 . 8 . 9 . 10 ___ **NP**

Some people have said I am responsible. I easily see what is illogical because I am analytical. I gather all the information I can and express my thoughts rationally. I am present in the moment and act respectfully. I think things through and show consideration. **Adult**

1 . 2 . 3 . 4 . 5 . 6 . 7 . 8 . 9 . 10 ___ **AD**

Some people have said I am carefree. I easily feel optimistic and happy, and can be charmingly persuasive. I am curious inventive, competitive, and/or playful. I live actively and enjoy showing affection. Io can act on impulse. **Spontaneous Child**

1 . 2 . 3 . 4 . 5 . 6 . 7 . 8 . 9 . 10 ___ **SC**

Some people have said I am sensitive. I easily feel defensive and apologize. I reflect a lot and can be tearful. I enjoy spending time alone and I am comfortable being quite. I feel overwhelmed and disengage. **Withdrawn Child**

1 . 2 . 3 . 4 . 5 . 6 . 7 . 8 . 9 . 10 ___ **WC**

Some people have said I am reactive. I easily see when things are places in my way, and say when these make me annoyed or frustrated. I believe I have to defend and protect myself when needed. I use strong language to show the intensity of what I feel. **Angry Child**

1 . 2 . 3 . 4 . 5 . 6 . 7 . 8 . 9 . 10 ___ **AC**

Some people have said I am self-assured. I easily see my own goodness and know where I'm going with myself. I live by setting meaningful objectives, and work to achieve them. I am the kind of person I want to be. **Self Esteem**

1 . 2 . 3 . 4 . 5 . 6 . 7 . 8 . 9 . 10 ___ **SE**

Optimal Range **Population Average**

Going Beyond the Call

Going Beyond the Call reprints with licensed permission by Verbal Aikido Inc.

TRANSACTIONAL ANALYSIS

"The unit of social intercourse is called a transaction. When two or more people encounter each other, sooner or later one of them will speak or give some other indication of acknowledging the presence of the others. This is called the transactional stimulus. Another person will then say or do something which is in some way related to the stimulus, and that is called the transactional response." This statement from Dr. Berne sets the stage for us to discuss Transactional Analysis.

Now that we understand the Ego States, we can begin to watch for patterns in others and analyze how they begin or respond to communication exchanges, especially emotionalized ones. As public safety professionals, being able to assess the Ego State you are faced with can aid your ability to manage your own reactions and communicate more effectively to avoid escalation. You will also avoid being triggered and with practice, gain competence in redirecting the conversation to an adult state using the tactics we will share as you. Just think of the escalations you can avoid, not to mention less paperwork! We will share some the predictable patterns of exchange, as well as the typical unpredictable ones. For each, how we initiate the communication has great bearing on how people respond. These Ego State responses are easy to hear when we pay attention. Verbal Aikido's James MacNeil has a great acronym for this called:

E.A.G.E.R. •
The Ego-state Addressed is Generally the Ego-state that Responds

When we speak to another from a parent state (without escalated emotion) we predictably get a parent state back, not necessarily the same parent tone as you presented, but a parent, nonetheless. As example.

PREDICTABLE	*PREDICTABLE*	*PREDICTABLE*
EGO STATE TO STATE	**PARENT TO CHILD**	**CHILD TO PARENT**

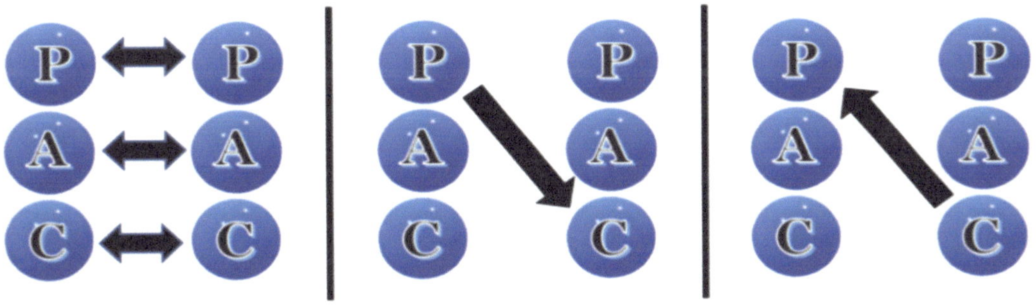

PARENT TO PARENT

You: **"Did you see that crappy coaching call on Johnny?"**

Them: **"YEAH, what an idiot!" (CP) or "I suppose, but that umpire has been distracted since his wife had the baby, he must be exhausted and not paying close attention to the game." (NP)**

PARENT TO CHILD

You: **"If you bought your kid the right weighted bat I bet he'd actually hit the ball rather than foul all the time!" (CP)** (Schooling/talking down to another)

Them: **"Mind you own business, and focus on your own kid, we can't all afford. The fancy equipment you get, you're just a pain in all our butts. No one likes you" (AC)**,(Defensive/bullying/lashing out)

CHILD TO PARENT

You: **"Why does that umpire hate my kid? He's always calling fair balls foul. He never gives Johnny a break; it's so unfair." (WC) (**Whiny, pouty, victim based)

Them: "You are right, it's unfair and it is harming our team's score, I am happy to go with you and give that umpire a piece of my mind (CP) (Wants to school the Ump and fix your problem) or "Oh you poor thing," your son is going to be in a terrible mood on the way home. Let me give you a number of a hitting coach we use. She is so awesome with kids, and she could help Johnny, so he isn't so close to the foul line to avoid these bad calls." (NP) (wants to sooth or calm the angered emotion and be helpful with finding a solution)

You can practice these scenarios to get comfortable with the concept, or simply think about a few recent conversations and consider where you started the conversation from and what ego state the reply came back as. ***How did you start? How did they reply?***

EGO STATE START: ______________________________

EGO STATE RESPONSE: ______________________________

EGO STATE START: ______________________________

EGO STATE RESPONSE: ______________________________

EGO STATE START: ______________________________

EGO STATE RESPONSE: ______________________________

EGO STATE START: ______________________________

EGO STATE RESPONSE: ______________________________

The other scenario you may find is when the response you expected is not what you were consciously or subconsciously seeking, and it will catch your internal awareness off guard.

CROSSED TRANSACTIONS		
Adult to Adult EGO seeks dominance so response is Critical Parent to Child.	Parent to Parent EGO seeks agreement to avoid escalating emotions or nurturing so response is Adult	Adult to Adult Ego seeks logic and reason but met with either Parent or Child States

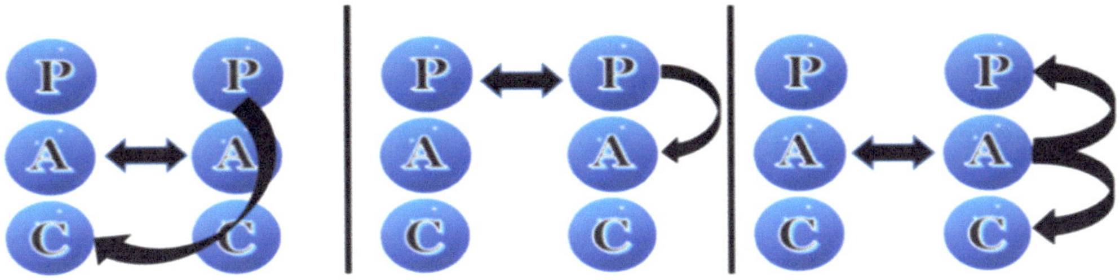

P P A A C C | P P A A C C | P P A A C C

ADULT TO ADULT ATTEMPT

You: **"I'm not sure that call was right. Hey Jane, can I see that footage to see if we should challenge that foul call?"**

Them: **"Geez Tom, you have to micromanage every darn game? This isn't the major leagues dude, just leave well enough alone and let the kids play." (CP to CP)**
(This response belittles your reasonable request to analyze the film before taking another step and tries to dismiss you and 'put you in your place' with sarcasm)

PARENT TO PARENT ATTEMPT

You: **"Why does that umpire hate my kid? He's always calling fair balls foul. He**

never gives Johnny a break; it's so unfair." (WC) (Whinny, pouty, victimized)

Them: **"I can understand how you may see that as a bad call from your angle. How about we go look at the filmed version and see whether there is a legitimate error. (A)** (Respects the point of view, so meets them where they are at, then redirects to a logical, fair option and invites them to join them in an adult state.)

ADULT TO ADULT ATTEMPT

You: **"I'm not sure that call was right. Hey Jane, can I see that footage to see if we should challenge that foul call?"**

Them: **"Oh here we go, the major league scout is in the house!" (A or C)**
(Pending body language and tone this could be criticizing and condemning, or it could be teasing and playful.)

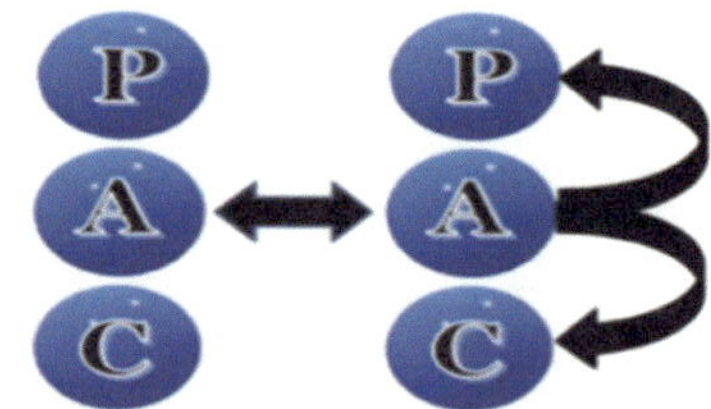

ULTERIOR
Adult to Adult Stimulated, and either child or parent state replies with ulterior motive to suck you into a drama or script.

There are also ulterior transactions where the responder wants to lead your conversation to a certain place surreptitiously. To feel you out, instigate a certain outcome, or push buttons to suck you into a drama, game, or script they are running. This is not always conscious, but when you hear it from now on, you will catch it faster.

ADULT TO ADULT ATTEMPT

You: **"I'm not sure that call was right. Hey Jane, can I see that footage to see if we should challenge that foul call?"**

Them: **Nudges your arm" … "I'd rather like to see footage of Jane, wouldn't you?"**

You: **(responds as child state) "who wouldn't! (wink)." Joined a "we have a secret pact club game."**

Them: **Chuckles and winks back (happy you joined his game).**

OR

You: **(responds as CP) "NO, what's wrong with you? That Gerry's wife, show some respect." (now talking down to an inappropriate child)**

Them: **"I was JUST kidding, don't be such a stick in the mud, Mr. Pious."** (Changed from spontaneous and playful to an angry child state).

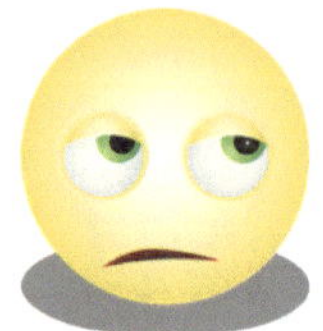

Certain Ego States tend to irritate us or push our emotional triggers more than others. We can often trace this back to unfavorable exchanges with parents or siblings.

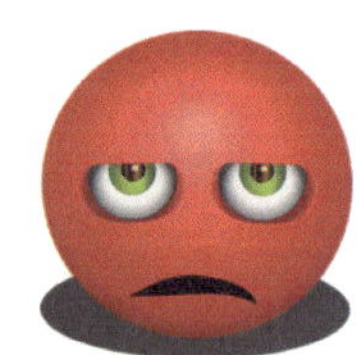

Go over the descriptive chart of Ego State traits and consider the following. Which Ego State irritates you the most?

____

Who in your close circle displays the Ego States that irritate you? What sort of repetitive arguments have you had with this person? Will you attempt to turn the next one using Adult Ego State comebacks now?

____

____

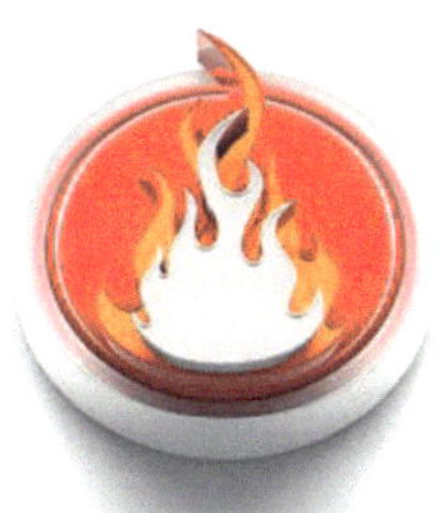

These higher response activators are your **HOT BUTTONS!** Being aware of what types of body mannerisms, tones, and ego state responses will trigger your emotional reactivity is key for a pre-escalation mindset and strategic communication perspective.

Consider practicing new approaches to gain better responses.

Typical sentence, phrase, or tone that seems to provoke a communication response I don't like.

How will I change my approach to get a better response?
If that doesn't work, what is my back up approach?

One of our interaction sessions in workshops focuses on how to demolish hot buttons in 30 minutes. It is a lot of fun to demonstrate and have participant's practice. If you haven't booked a seat in one of our two days workshops, then connect with us for extra tactics only available in classes.

GBTC911.COM ***GoingBeyondTheCall.com***

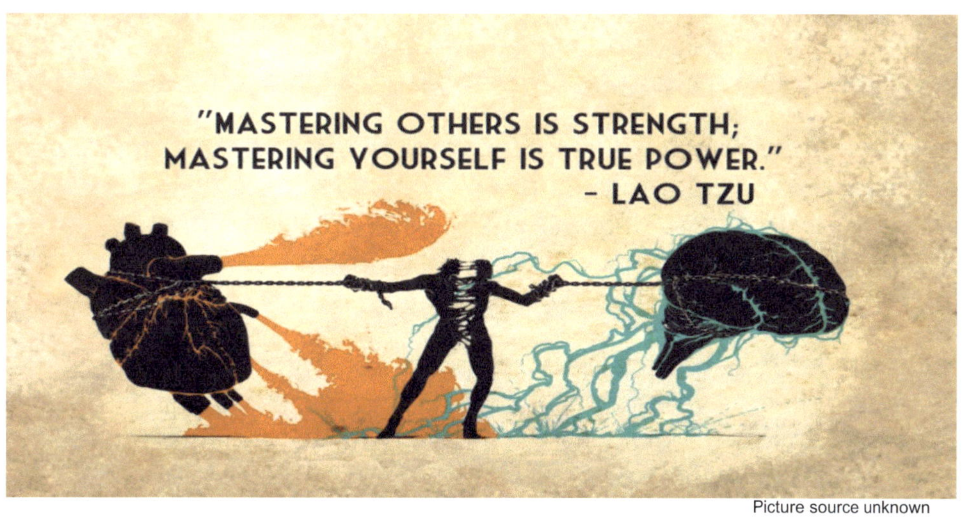

Picture source unknown

LIFE POSITIONS – READ CHAPTER 20

Dr. Thomas Harris, a student of Dr. Eric Berne describes four life positions. ***"Within the earliest months and sometimes later, a central emotional position is frequently established ... it becomes the primary position to which that individual will tend to return automatically for the rest of his or her days. This, in turn, may constitute either the primary safeguard or the major vulnerability of his or her life. Whenever the central emotional position is painful ... the individual may spend his whole life defending himself against it, again using conscious, preconscious, and unconscious devices whose aim it is to avoid this pain-filled central position. Kubie then raises the question as to whether or not these positions are alterable later in life. I believe they are. Although the early experiences which culminated in the position cannot be erased, I believe the early positions can be changed. What was once decided can be undecided." ~ Dr. Thomas Harris, author of I'm OK; You're OK."***

YOU ARE OKAY WITH ME

I AM NOT OKAY WITH ME | I AM OKAY WITH ME

I AM NOT OKAY YOU ARE OKAY DEPRESSIVE POSITION "GET AWAY FROM" HELPLESS	I AM OKAY YOU ARE OKAY HEALTHY POSITION "GET ON WITH" HAPPY
I AM NOT OKAY YOU ARE NOT OKAY POSITION OF DESPAIR "GO NOWHERE" HOPELESS	I AM OKAY YOU ARE NOT OKAY ARROGANT/PARANOID POSITION "GET RID OF" ANGRY

YOU ARE NOT OKAY WITH ME

Where are you on this chart?

____

____

____

____

____

____

The first three positions are primarily developed by the circumstances of our upbringing and by the age of three most have adopted a general belief of position one "I am not okay, you are okay" as we are under a barrage of "wrong" and "no" from our parental influences.

Sadly, the second and third positions "I'm not okay, you're not okay" and "I'm okay, you're not okay" come from abusive, highly restrictive, or traumatic experiences where loving parental 'strokes' are missing or unhealthy. The fourth position "I'm okay, you're okay" is one of choices and developed conscious beliefs and actions grown from our emotional intelligence.

As we develop our Adult Ego State, gain independence and self-regard from new accomplishments, and receive 'strokes' from new sources, many shift to position four, "I'm okay, You're okay". For some, this may not happen until further independence occurs in adulthood, for others the shift is never made.

STROKES

We all have a basic human desire to be acknowledged and seek out "stokes" to reinforce how we feel about ourselves. While the desire for positive strokes is strong when they are not available, we will act in a manner that gains negative strokes. The absence of strokes is the most harmful thing to the human psyche. This is why time-outs in another room away from the family or activity work, or why having your phone call or text ignored hurts so much. It is also why solitary confinement is so powerful in our prison system.

Strokes Can be Wanted or Unwanted

Strokes which are positive in nature are not necessarily wanted by any one specific person. Strokes can be Physical, Verbal, or Non-verbal (Action Strokes):

- Physical strokes can be simple touch, hugs, kisses, caresses, back rubs, being held, holding hands.
- Verbal strokes can be about a person's looks, clothing, intelligence, generosity, creativity, elegance, wisdom, dignity, leadership ability, tact, warmth, energy, taste, honesty, or any attribute a person possesses.
- Action strokes are non-verbal forms of recognition like listening empathizing, or actively liking or loving someone.

Think about each stroke type in the chart below and provide an example of when you have experienced each stoke; also, when you have dished each one out to another person close to you.

____

____

____

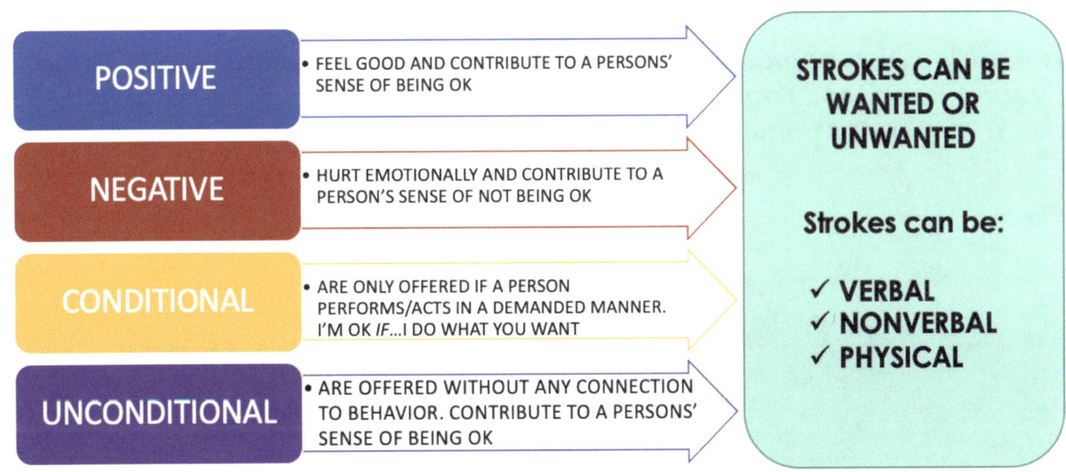

GAMES PEOPLE PLAY 1.5-hour Audible book reading on YouTube: https://www.youtube.com/watch?v=reCfhZSLC_k

Games People Play: The Psychology of Human Relationships is a bestselling book on the various aspects of social interactions and human relationships. It was authored Eric Berne who said, "A game us an ongoing series of complementary ulterior transactions progressing to a well-defined, predictable outcome. Descriptively, it is a recuring set of transactions with a concealed motivation, or gimmick. Games are learned patterns of behavior, and most people play a small number of favorite games with a range of different people and in varying intensities."

We may not consider our learned interaction and conversational behavior patterns and are quite that predictable but studying some of the games listed will give you some insight on where you may be party to an interactive game. Games are played with different people with various intensities, how we interact with a contentious family member will be different that how we communicate with a superior we dislike. Most games are not intent on positive relationship outcomes, an example for children would be the "mine is better than yours" exchanges. Games most often come from a critical parent to child Ego State and avoid the equality and reasonableness of the Adult.

COMMON GAMES INCLUDE:

Game	Description	Real benefit
Stop me if you can	Damaging activity, for example using drugs.	Gets attention, avoids responsibility
Blemish	Finding fault with others. Being as picky as necessary	Distracts attention from self
Clever me	Boasting about what you have done	Get attention, sympathy, admiration
Courtroom	Describe 'logically' how I am right and others are wrong	Get support, sympathy and absolution
If it weren't for you	Blaming others for your non-achievements	Absolution of guilt
I'm only trying to help	Offering help then complaining when it is not accepted	Controlling others
Let's you and him fight	Get others to fight for you	Control of others, share of blame, friendship
Look how hard I've tried	Put in lots of effort that intentionally does not succeed.	Absolves oneself from responsibility.
Now I've got you (you son of a bitch)	Vents rage on someone and blames them for it	Displaces anger. Absolves responsibility
Poor me	Display self as unlucky and helpless	Sympathy and support
See what you made me do	Blaming others for one's own problems	Absolution of responsibility, instilling guilt
Honestly	Making empty promises	Getting one's way in the short-term
Uproar	Violent argument with deliberate pressing of hot buttons	Sustain attention, venting and displacing anger
Yes but...	Providing objections to refuse help	Maintenance of attention and control
Wooden leg	Acquire a handicap, real or imagined and ham it up	Sympathy, avoidance of responsibility

**Source: ChangingMinds.org*

Who in your life play games with you? Who do you play games with? Reflect on where your games took root in childhood and what attention, or action was the incentive to play your game(s). Do they still serve you well?

DRAMA TRIANGLE

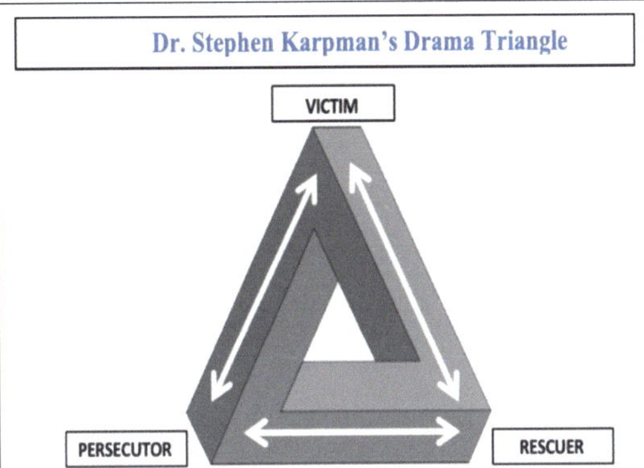

When one of these games triggers us in the right way or by the right person, we will jump on the Drama Triangle at some base point with various levels of intensity.

Who in your life starts out as a:

Victim: ___________________________

Rescuer:___________________________

Persecutor: ____________________

What is your starting point most often?

____

PERSECUTOR	VICTIM	RESCUER
I am better than you I discount you I blame you I put you down	I can't I am no good Self-pity Poor me I have no idea	You need me You can't I know better than you You're lacking
	DESCRIBED AS	
Aggressive Angers easy Judgmental	Helpless Complains of unmet needs Downtrodden	Over-helpful Self-sacrificing Needs to be needed
	TYPES OF STATEMENTS	
It's your fault! What were you thinking?" Why did you do that? What's your problem?	I'm not responsible! I don't know what to do. Why is this happening to me? No one likes me!	Let me help you! I will do that for you. I feel bad for you. You'll be fine, I'm here.
	DISCOUNTING ASPECT	
Discounts others value and worthiness. Tends to put people down or "put them in their place." Views others as one down from them and "Not OK." In extremes they may bully, belittle and become emotionally abusive.	Discounts themselves, he or she puts themselves in a one down position and "Not OK." Common for the victim to seek out a persecutor to put them down and push them around as they feel they deserve it. May also search for rescuers who will offer help and confirm the victim's inner belief that they just cannot cope well on their own. Often an adapted child mindset of where "it's not fair," "it's not my fault," finding blame outside of themselves. In the extreme these all lead to relationship draining constant drama.	Discounts another's ability to think for themselves or show initiative. Tends to believe you do not act in your own best interest. Sees others as "Not OK" and from a one down position. Feel's their offer of help can move them one up to better life position. In extremes, they can be intrusive or see themselves as martyrs and will attract victims to them.

For those who do not believe they enter the Drama Triangle, I have one word … Denial. Those that say, "I don't have any drama," see their behavior pattern as I am right, and you or your drama is wrong. That is a persecutor role. Those that say, "I don't cause or participate in the drama," are saying they are the rescuer in this situation. Those that feel "I have no drama, it is what it is, it's out of my hands" when they are unsatisfied are coming from a victim role. If you are resistant and stubborn with this assessment, you are missing out on an opportunity to heal a cyclical conversation pattern with one or more people in your life. A pattern that likely does not serve you well and leaves you frustrated.

When I am around this person, I feel this starting position on the drama triangle, e.g. When I am around my older brother I feel victim to his persecutor role, although I have been his rescuer and persecutor as well.

____

____

POWER COMMUNICATIONS - Read Chapter 12

Why it's important to balance heart and mind

RAPPORT is the invisible bridge between two souls. Whether you are trying to build a new relationship or you want someone to cooperate with you, it starts with how you are perceived. As much as your situational awareness is turned up inspecting them, they too are taking in your body language, words, tone, pitch, volume, and vibe. You cannot change anyone else, but you can change yourself.

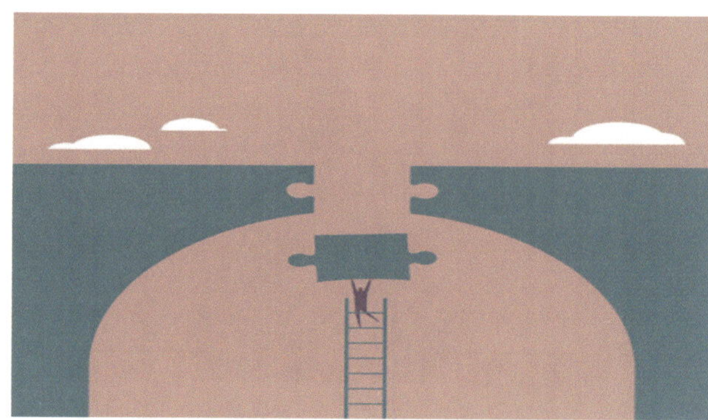

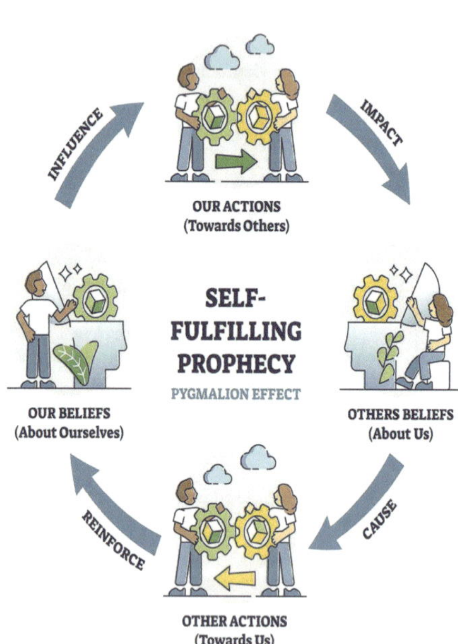

Consider your resonance in self-projection. The way we are treated is often based on how we project ourselves to be treated. There is some intelligence behind the "fake it till you make it" or "dress for the job you want not the job you have," style statements. While I would not advocate trying to be someone completely fake (people will see thought that), we often fail to consider what parts of ourselves we want to grow and project to the world and what we will be remembered for.

If you show up with a wrinkled, sloppy uniform, a scowling face, a gruff vocal start, and expect to be respected just because you are in a uniform, you should not be surprised if you do not get what you are looking for. Then you get upset at the lack of respect, so you act in a way that furthers the disconnect between the rapport we expected from someone and what we get. In this example you can see the self-fulfilling prophecy in full effect.

Learn to present yourself with calm, safe, approachable (but alert) presence and you will have far fewer escalated situations you then have to de-escalate. You don't have to like them, love them, or even have sympathy for them. An empathetic approach that meets them where they are at and influences them to the best possible option for all involved is the best pre-escalation approach when safety is not a primary concern. Sometimes creating an "Alter Ego" can help you develop the new persona you wish to emulate. Like a superhero putting on their costume, you step into the envisioned role until it naturally blends with your ideal self-perception and helps change your self-fulfilling prophecy.

WATCH: THE ALTER EGO EFFECT by Todd Herman https://youtu.be/mETY4zT3ZNg

Being consistent and congruent in your message from body language, vocalization, and the words used is the beginning of rapport building. When we are consistent and congruent, we are powerful communicators.

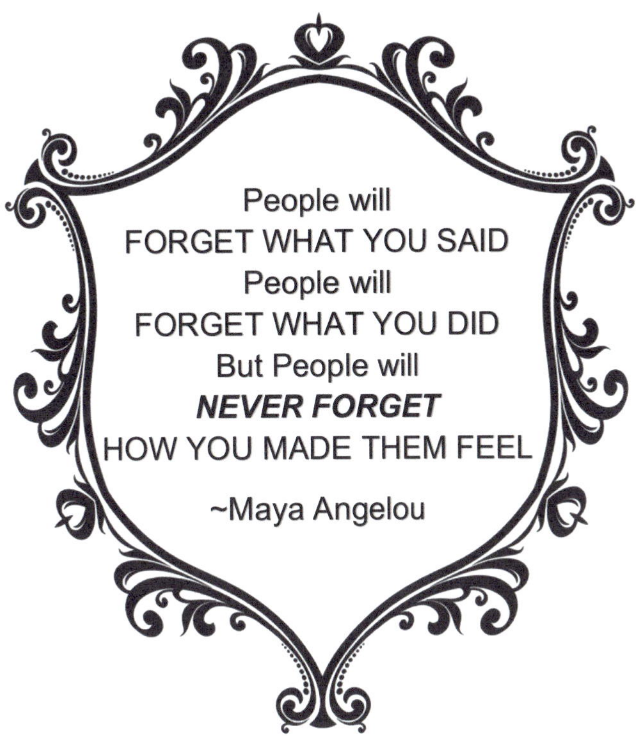

It takes less than a tenth of a second for our RAS to determine a threat, after this, you will have formed a solid impression within 3-7 seconds. The brain is judging trustworthiness, status, and attractiveness and this is where all our implicit and explicit biases come into play. It is also where you may face bias from the opposing person from their own experiences, as well as fears infused by media, environmental, and generational trauma.

The limbic (emotional center) will dominate our initial impressions blindly if we do not consciously present ourselves and challenge our thinking.

When we take corrective action with mindful thinking and intentional presence, we are offering the counter person unconscious and open consideration in our facial expressions, body language, and verbal use. As we recall from earlier, building trust is the first goal to aim for. The only way to sway the pre-loaded escalation game is to stop the cycle within yourself and invite others to join you in adult-to-adult ego state communication.

Write about when your initial impression about someone was completely off base once you got to know them. Consider a positive to negative and a negative to positive experience.

RECEPTIVE INFLUENCE

Verbal Aikido continues to power our communication strategies as the alignment between this particular marital art and challenging communication exchanges fits. We want to receive the energy (meet them where they are at), redirect the energy (leaving emotions aside, redirect the energy to an adult-to-adult ego state exchange), and maintain an alert and adaptable stance while emitting a safe strength, calm energy, and mindful interaction.

When it comes to questioning an emotionalized person, a Verbal Aikido question is the master move for maintaining your adaptive communication balance. Master move questions are information seeking questions, based on what the other person has just said, directed towards your objective. It is not a closed question (yes or no answers), it is not an open question (that can lead you way off track), think of it as an open-directive question. It is best accomplished when you have a communication objective in mind before you begin.

Information seeking question:

The value in this is to engage the adult ego state. No matter how high the emotion is, every time you use this move you invite them into an adult-to-adult ego state conversation. Provoking the other person to the best possible non-emotionally controlled version of themselves. Then slowly lessening the emotion and working to keep the remaining conversation where it is most effective for the best overall outcome for all involved.

Mindful listening:

Next, based on what the other person has just said, I am leading and influencing the direction of the conversation or questioning. Why is that important? Based on what they've just said they have unconsciously put information out there, so it's fair play. You are letting them know, they are heard, understood accepted and respected. You have actively listened and are using that insight to continue the direction of the conversation. There's nothing more honoring than asking an information seeking question based on what another person has just said to you. It's the ultimate sign you have listened. But it's not just honoring them directionless, we are asking all those cascading questions that are directing us to our situational objective, which we have identified at the beginning of the conversation.

Ethical Influence:

It is constantly influencing and ethically moving towards the conclusion of the best possible outcome for all involved. It's not a technique that is finite in its options; there is a lot of ways that you can ask the same forms of questions. Now, let's be real, in some cases that outcome will still have detrimental aspects for someone, whether it is going to jail, recognizing a need for marriage counselling, or identifying an addiction in a peer or close friend. However, the win-win victory is you got there without inflaming the situation further with emotional escalation that could have made the outcome worse for both, or, all of you.

VERBAL AIKIDO QUESTIONING:

The questioning format is clarifying the why of the conversation (set the stage) and, when this is a peer or personal exchange that can be delayed, ask for agreement on timing (rite of passage). Then initiate by asking an open-directed question, consider the recipient statement and follow by a clarifying statement, then repeat. This gives the person a clear feeling that they have been heard. You catch their response where it was sent, adapt the verbal aikido stance of adult-to-adult ego state before sending back the next directive question. Use a clarifying statement to show attentive listening and where appropriate to provide an empathetic vibe.

As an example, "*tell me what happened*" is a broad open-ended question, sometimes helpful if you want a lot of background but it opens the flood gates on emotions and past influences. Better to use the open-ended near the end of a conversation when you have built some rapport and want to capture anything else that might further your interest in the subject matter at hand. Therefore, "tell me what happened between ____ and ____ on this date" is a more open-directed question.

Strategic empathy added into the questioning sequence is a chance to deepen rapport. As example you could say, "I hear where you're coming from", "it seems very important from your perspective", or "I agree it would be good to address that issue." This will show empathy without sympathy and still maintain an adult-to-adult ego state stance.

Utilizing honoring words, we can keep them in the adult ego state easier by using these strategic choices of words and matching and mirroring some of their body language and verbal cues. When someone is communicated to in a manner that they feel heard, understood, accepted, and respected, a rapport bridge is quickly built. As an example, you could ask "tell me what happened" which may evoke a parent ego state to child ego state response pending the situation. Or you could ask "would you please share your perspective on ________ (this)" using a collaborative tone. The words "*please share your perspective on…*" is more honoring than saying, "*tell me about,*" and it is more apt to evoke an adult-to-adult conversation.

Redirects are best when begun with clarifying aspects to confirm you were listening. As example, saying "so I hear what you're saying is …, (*attentive listening by clarifying a detail or two*), "I agree with this perspective", (*empathetic alignment*) or "I understood something different, may I clarify a couple of things, or may I share my perspective?" (*Respectful and collaborative disagreement*).

Part of rapport building is setting the stage first. Questions without a context are a crime. If you ask a question and don't let a person know why you are asking the questions, they may be uncomfortable or defensive and refuse to respond or create a more challenging escalated exchange.

This questioning technique is extremely beneficial in personal relationships as well as with peers and the community you serve. If you receive a call from a casual friend and they say, "what are you doing Saturday?" many of us have learned to reply, "why are you asking?"

We want to understand the context first before opening ourselves up to something we don't want to do or respond to.
That is the same for any questions where we may feel we have to be a little vulnerable, exposed, or potentially guarded. In a work context we want to avoid interacting and questioning in a way that provokes fear, pride, or confusion as that leads to emotionalized responsiveness. Therefore, with any difficult or emotionalized conversation, we want to ensure we prepare our receiver by setting the stage and providing a why first.

- *"I would like to understand what happened here today; would you share your perspective on…?"*
- *"I have noticed you seem really down lately. I'm not sure what I can do to help, but I would sure like to listen and ensure you know you have someone trusted to talk to."*
- *"I feel like our finances are getting a little away from us. When the kids go to sleep tonight can we sit and go over our budget?"*
- *"While I appreciate you want to protect me from the crap you deal with at work, you seem very distant lately. I'd like to have a conversation about how we can connect better on your next days off rotation."*

Can someone think of a situation you have experienced that blew way out of hand because the questioning approach put you or the other person on guard and it got ugly from there?

____

____

____

____

____

Write out two or three scenarios where you could use this questioning technique.

____

____

____

The golden rule is common and prominent in every religion, spiritual group, and people around the world. It is a message of intentional, purposeful action that gives focus to our behavior in any interaction."
~ Deirdre von Krauskopf

Do unto Others as you would have them do unto You.

What does respect mean to you?

____

____

____

Currently, is it outward facing? Meaning do you give it before you expect it? Or is it inward facing and expected before it is given?

____

____

____

WRAP-UP ... QUESTION / EXAMPLES

1. It would be so helpful to understand how this all started, would you share that with me?
2. So, if I understand you correctly (repeat back their message)
3. Seek clarification if their words or body language informs you missed something.
4. Ask open directed questions, "you mentioned _______ or I believe I understand this part, I am curious about (such and such)," a leading question to gain the information you seek.
5. When they finish and you have clarified always ask "is there anything else that would help me understand _____________?"
6. Empathize … "I understand that must have made you angry." I'm sorry you had that experience." "I wish there was a better outcome for you." Without sympathy or acceptance.
7. Let's work together to find the best possible outcome for this situation."
8. Strike the right CHORD! Do you mind if I communicate honestly, openly, respectfully, and directly with you on this topic?"
9. Mirror and match their body language, tonality, words choices (audible, verbal, or feeling words) when appropriate and authentic to do so. They will pick up on inauthentic actions.
10. Maintain open (but ready) posturing and active listening gestures.
11. If they have radically different values than you, listen with curiosity not judgement (it will help maintain your rapport vibe). "I see, I hadn't considered (__) that perspective, thank you for sharing.

What questions can you think about reframing to entice a more respectful, adult to adult, conversation?

____

____

____

____

MANAGING DIFFICULT CONVERSATIONS

READ Chapter 12

Too often our society promotes the false idea that you are either powerful or you are weak, you are a winner or a loser, you are the victor or the victim; therefore, you must choose a side. Interactions where one side has the "power" to dominate with authoritative control, perceived prestige and wealth makes the other side feel quite weak and disempowered. When one reacts from a disempowered state, often fear, pride or confusion leads the response. As we learned in the previous chapter, when negative and emotionalized triggers are in play, our reasoning and logic centers are not being utilized fully.

If that feeling of human suppression becomes a predominant thought, it becomes easier to understand the screams of defiance within groups, as well as why it quickly spreads. From a fear state, people can quickly escalate within themselves. Every negative, horrifying, devastating event seen or heard about gets piled on their emotional memory reaction.

This triggers a fear-based response against those in the perceived power position; they react in whatever small way they can within their circle of control. This the birthplace of riots, criminal responses and life altering poor choices and actions. The same type of trigger for a perceived "play" for power and control is seen in bullies and abusers. They find someone or someway to exert power over others, so they feel less a victim, less a "loser," and less diminished in that moment. They are trying to dominate in some small way to challenge perceived threat.

As a public safety professional, knowing this gives you the opportunity to adjust your approach, ***if safe to do so***. Shifting from a physical and verbal power-based authority to using powerful communications tactics allows you to meet people where they are, and to seek common ground. When you interact with someone whose hackles are already up, they may already be triggered by the moment that caused your call. As you approach the scene, you are like a spark approaching an incendiary device. Your very presence can invoke fear, pride, or confusion in others, due to their emotionally driven need to feel some power in the situation.

A further advantage of using this tactic is self-preservation. If we can alter our perspective to recognize the aggressive antics of someone who is acting out as a 5-year-old child, we can maintain power without flexing our outward muscles. We have the intelligence to understand we are the adult in the situation while others around us throw a temper tantrum. Everything can be captured in an instant, clipped for the most dramatic impact, and viral before proper context can be verified. With social media, that facts are not relevant and the only thing that matters is the dramatic spin.

It may seem odd or contrived to start a difficult conversation with a communication objective but doing so primes us to approach, interact, manage, and influence from a position of calm, safe, strength. We wouldn't go into a take down without having a clear objective and communicating with social/emotional underpinning is just as much a powder keg potential. Our person difficult conversations are the same. We need to understand our compelling objective and our negotiating parameters for a win-win outcome. *For every difficult personal conversation have you considered your "Worst Case Scenario" you can live with?*

"Difficult People" think we're "Difficult People" The other person:

Feels they are being reasonable	Feels they are being fair	Hates being interrupted
Cannot hear when they do not feel heard	Doesn't understand why you don't see things from their perspective	Has fears, needs, frustrations & insights, you will never know about
Feels their irrational behavior is justified	Likely feels you're the "bad guy"	Interprets "I know" as "I'm not listening to you"
Gets bored when you talk too long	Can't read your mind	Feels the need to repeat themselves when they don't feel heard

Questions that keep you on track without becoming emotionally reactive help with the above.

"If I understand you correctly, you said**______________________________**

In personal relationships, a great counter statement asks permission to share countering views. It can also keep you in check to truly listen until the other person feels heard. Only if you have done a good job managing yourself up to this point understand that most objections are rarely firm. They are usually a push-back tactic … so stop pushing – start listening.

OBJECTION

OK

I happen to have a different opinion on the subject.
Would you care to hear it? Or may I share a different viewpoint?

What challenging conversation have you been putting off that you would like to try these tactics with?

____

____

____

____

____

What is your conversational objective? What are you willing to concede for a harmonious outcome?

____

____

____

PSYCHOLOGICAL AIR

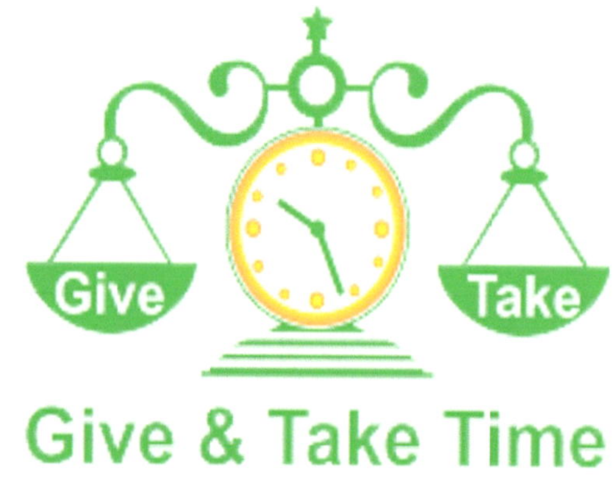

Psychological Air is the principle which raises awareness of the need to allow a natural flow of "give" and "take" within an interaction. Everybody needs, psychologically, to hear and be heard. An individual is likely to become open to "respectfully listen" after they feel heard, accepted, valued, empathized with, and understood. People can only inhale (hear) for so long and then they need to exhale (be heard).

When you begin a conversation, know that the other person's psychological air, like a cup, may be full. In today's fast paced society, the saying "*their cup runneth over*" is a good phrase to keep in mind.

Be prepared that the first few times you try this with someone that has not felt heard in the past that they may run on, and on. If that is the case, prepare the person and let them know you want to try a new communication tactic you learned. Have an agreed upon method to interject or allow each other to jot notes so they can come back to counter points when the other person ends. After a few times you will both be better at the give and take time frame. Future challenging conversations will go much smoother.

____

____

____

____

____

KEY POINTS:

1. When you begin a conversation, understand that their mind may be racing with 12 other issues occurring in their life at that moment. Understand that a person has a full cup much of the time, therefore, it is suggested to start the conversation with an information seeking question.

2. When we ask an information-seeking question we will enable the other person to exhale and thereby create the psychological room for new ideas.

3. When a person won't stop talking, they may feel that you have not understood them. One strategy to deal with this is to ask permission to restate what they are saying along the way, so that they know you want to understand what they are saying.

4. Pace your conversation to ensure you are not dominating the talk and allowing the flow to enable the emptying of the other person's cup.

PSYCHOLOGICAL COMMUNICATION TACTICS – READ CHAPTER 17

The last aspect to consider is communication tactics that facilitate deepening conversations. If you ask psychologists and psychotherapists, they will say everything that is said, is said for a reason. So, if somebody says something, not only is it technically on the table for conversation, but it is also intentionally on the table, even if subconsciously. There may be some exceptions, but this is generally a scientifically validated way to look at it. In addition to the words, the method of conveying the message have been offered from a body language, tone, pitch, pace, and volume standpoint. If I ask, "How are you doing?" and you reply, "Fine," in a manner that raises my eyebrows, I have been offered the opportunity to say, "Well I heard the word 'fine,' but I'm not feeling that from you. Would you like to talk?" The door to communication has been cracked, and if our rapport is good, you may choose to open up further.

The strategy is useful in pre-escalation rapport building when dealing with the public; however, it is absolutely gold when used in your personal relationships. You can wait for that simmering hint of discontent to become more overt, or you can choose to jump on the hint you were offered and tackle the emotion before it grows. When we consider these moments in a manner where we respect the invitation to dive deeper and use the moment to serve the relationship, we have learned the secrets of receptivity.

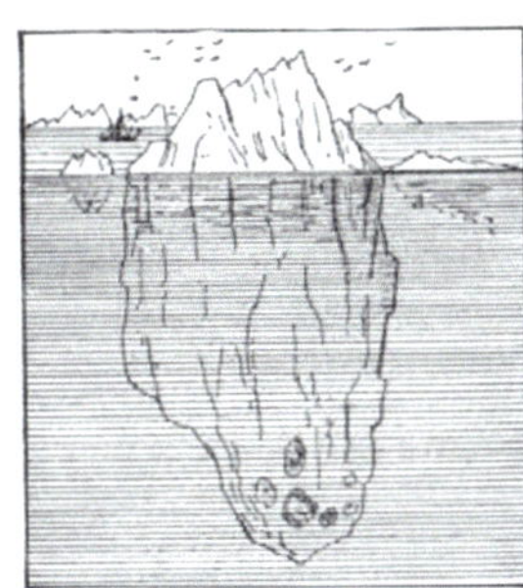

Think of every word, the person's body language and tonality as the tip of an iceberg. All of these are invitations to deepen an interaction. Be prepared when you take the next step; you want both of you to be able and willing to invest in the time that may come next. By diving deeper, we may find something that would be very valuable to our conversation or our overall relationship. It could resolve a meaningful objective or work towards a stronger rapport. Setting the stage for the right time and place becomes a critical step before moving forward.

EVERY WORD IS LIKE THE TIP OF AN ICEBERG.

Think of a conversation where you know what was said was completely contrary to what you heard and received from the underpinning body language, words, and verbal cues? Did you confront the fact or chose to ignore it? Will you use these tactics to challenge future situations like these?

____

____

____

____

____

____

EVERY SENTENCE IS LIKE A DOOR

Our next psychological communication tactic comes from a slightly subtle tell people tend to have. Imagine that every word is a door. Some doors are wide open, some are closed, and some are squeaky.

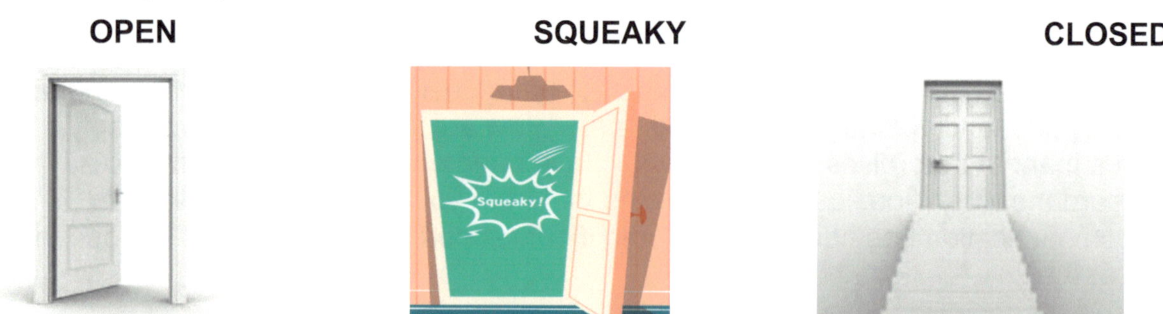

Most doors are wide open, since almost everything spoken is said for a reason. Once it is on the table, it is fair play. Some words are like squeaky doors, this is investigative gold, you know there's something there. You will hear it when a subtle sound emits after a word, and it draws out a little. Let's say you ask your significant other to go to a movie and mention the one you want to see. They reply, *"I guessssss,"* or *"if youuu want to."*

This is when someone puts something on the table, but they are not fully comfortable with it. They are seeking safety and comfort before they trust enough to open up. They are putting feelers out to see if you will treat their next words with respect. We can say, "I sensed a little more than what you said there. Would you help me understand what is behind the hesitancy?" Depending on the rapport between us and their feeling of safety, you may hear, "Okay, well the truth is…" and they begin to open up that they hate that type of movie.

In a questioning or investigative sense, you might say, "I hear from the way you sounded there that there is more you would like to share. I would really appreciate your further insight." Invite them to trust you by showing you were truly listening and interested in what they have to say.

Think of a time where the squeaky door happened, and you knew there was more but didn't know how to approach it. What will you do in the future?

____

____

When we use psychological communication tactics, we want to do so with authenticity so that everything they say can, and will, be used to SERVE THEM by moving towards the best possible solution for all involved.

If you use these tactics for manipulative purposes, you will get caught, at least subconsciously. Your intention will differ from your words and body language and on some level, they will pick it up an inauthentic vibe. Incongruency always shows, whether or not they know WHY they don't trust what you are saying is based on their level of self-development in this area.

ETHICS OF INFLUENCE

"Helping others across the threshold of making an informed decision in their own best interest." ~ Bob Sears

Bob Sears, an internationally renowned master sales coach, teaches ethical influence in the sales and marketing arena. When Deirdre heard him speak on a joint speaking tour, she was instigated to read more about the influence our social media, friends, and marketing conglomerates have over our everyday thinking.

It also had her aligning social psychology, neuroscience, and strategic communications in all her corporate courses. While a whole book and workshop could be dedicated to this subject alone, she wants to end our Going Beyond the Call workbook sharing the bridge between marketing and personal influence. How we can market ourselves to gain the best possible outcome for all involved by understanding some basics of human behavior influence.

Robert B Cialdini PhD, is a leading authority on influence and persuasion. He has written a number of books that provide the secret sauce of exceptional salespeople and integrated into all AI tracking, media, and print marketing. He has published a number of books aimed at marketing or look him up on YouTube for some of his presentations. You will never make a large purchase, or an impulse purchase the same naïve way again!

His tactics can also be very useful in strategic communications. When you hope to lead someone to a decision in the best interest of all involved, with minimum emotionalized escalation, your level of influence is a critical factor to success. There is good, bad, and downright nasty when it comes to influence and persuasion, so it is important to remain authentic. When you are not, you will be found out, perhaps not immediately; but definitely don't try this at home and hope to get away with the manipulative aspects of this science.

His original six principles are reciprocity, commitment/consistency, social proof, authority, liking, scarcity, and he later published a seventh principle of unity. Unity ties well into Maslow's hierarchy of needs in the power of belonging. The growth of online influencers has exploded this desire to fit into shared identities of those we feel are above us in the social hierarchy.

Have you ever bought something and felt you were "ripped off" after some time passed? Or felt you were 'suckered' into helping another when you really didn't want to?

____

____

____

____

1. Reciprocity: Give something to get a little something in return.

Cialdini's first principle of persuasion plays off the golden rule. As humans we are wired for cooperative exchange which means we like to return favors and pay back our debts. When we consistently focus our communications and presence to project a calm, safe, leader that is building towards rapport, the counterpart will find it difficult (subconsciously) to remain angry, belligerent, or overly emotional. It may take a while if they are really ramped up, but consistency of behavior, empathetic approach, meeting them where they are at, our adult ego state, body language, and approach will create incongruency to yours versus their emotional state and they will be driven to match you.

Think about a time where you felt obliged to give back, whether it was providing a more intimate bit of information about yourself or a helping hand. Write out the experience.

---

2. Consistency/Commitment: Humans generally strive to have their beliefs and commitments to be consistent with their values.

Who wants to be seen as scattered or unreliable? Generally, people have a deep need to be seen as consistent and reliable, especially when the context is important to them. If we can gain little commitments in communication, like someone's acceptance that we can communicate, honestly, openly, respectfully, and directly, we are influencing their subconscious to stay true to their word. When in a group setting and we gain that commitment, we actually influence the whole lot to help the person maintain their word.

Psychologically, the person we are influencing wishes to maintain their self-image and those around them will aid in maintaining the self-projection they have built up with those known to them. This is where you will see a friend or family member shift hostility towards you to helping you keep someone calm after the person has begun to cooperate and perhaps slips a little when triggered.

3. Social Proof: The need for validation

It can be summarized as safety in numbers. It is more powerful when someone is unsure of themselves and trying to fit in, or when we strive to be accepted into a group or image that appeals to us as similar to our social and self-image. There are numerous social psychology studies that example this phenomenon. You will likely have seen it in your social and peer groups when a majority of the group start to automatically mimic characteristics of the more valued in the social circle.

In conversational influence it can be utilized by inviting others into the conversation, or seeking positive agreement with gestures to concur, when you believe they will back your influence. "Hey, you don't want your friend to keep escalating this, blowing it up to the point they have to go to jail, right?! None of us want that!" (Look around seeking agreement and see how many will mimic your body language, mumble some type of alignment, or even speak up in agreement for the better outcome).

4. Authority: You will respect my authority!

There is definitely a time and place for an authoritative persona. Whether a first responder, boss, educational, or a medical professional, people will generally follow instructions of someone perceived to be the uniformed or expert authority in their field.
Heck, you can have a group of cop haters readily switch gears and accept instruction to move quickly in an indicated direction when a truck swerves into their protest path because their RAS alerts their lives are in danger. They will acquiesce to the known authority as it clicks as necessary in their subconscious. It works in a social contagion way as well. Look at the political separation between humans when a political race is on. The candidate may have little or no expertise in a particular matter being debated but folks will jump onto the us versus them and right versus wrong band wagon without independent research because of the perceived authority of a political figure.

Authority works best when we can influence another that we are working in their best interest as the expert that can help or hinder their life. Conversationally, we could have more power saying, “I could arrest you (or write you up) over this, but I would prefer to help you by working through this with as little pain/damage as possible. Would you please work with me to keep the outcome reasonable for both of us.” You have invited them to influence their own outcome, in their own best interest, even though it is clear you are in charge.

5. Liking: Relationships work better when you like each other.

The more you like someone, the more you'll be persuaded by them.
We are not talking about becoming besties but there is a science behind why good cop/bad cop works. When we feel someone is agreeable, nice, friendly, and likable we are more apt to lean in and be open and receptive to influence. Social science teaches us that we like those most like us, so making the effort to find mutual interests or values can be extremely valuable when we wish to influence someone.

Deirdre shares a powerful interactive lesson learned from her grandfather as a child and told in her book and class “UnQuiet Warrior.” He would say “*people are fascinating, if you look hard enough there is always something interesting to learn*.” Now his context was as a mayor making rounds to his constituents. It served him to remain agreeable to those who may be opposed to him in some way. It has driven Deirdre to find something to like about every person she meets. It may be nothing more than flattering their choice of clothing or the design on a tie. Yet, it will light up someone's eyes and create that moment of rapport because it was driven by authentically liking something about them.

6. Scarcity: The desire for items in short supply as they become more valuable.

In marketing it is the “last chance,” “almost sold out” allure that drives many impulse buys. In influential conversation it is the time available to maintain a positive conversational outcome. We have five more minutes to maintain the (outcome) discussed thus far or (worst scenario) will happen.

In personal relationships it can be a time limit on thinking things over before a more negative outcome is decided. With teenagers it can be "you have 15 minutes to clean your room, or you lose your phone for a day." Scarcity of time is as effective as scarcity of a sales item. The biggest challenge with this principle is authenticity, if you are going to threaten a worse outcome based on time you had better see it through. Consistency is king in this area.

7. **Unity: To invoke a group's traits, rituals, characteristics in attempt to form an immediate bond.**

Dr. Robert Cialdini states, "It's about the categories that individuals use to define themselves and their groups, as example, race, ethnicity, nationality, family, political, and religious affiliations. A key characteristic of these categories is that the members feel comfortably merged with the others. They are the categories in which the conduct of one member influences the self-esteem of other members. Simply put, "we," becomes the shared "me."

This is not always a great human drive as it is often used to instigate negative herding, in politics (to appeal to voter segments), social anarchists, cult leaders, as well as unscrupulous social marketing, or "influencers." It is an influential manner to create unity by invoking a group likes, traits, rituals, or characteristics in order to form a quick bond. Neurolinguistic Programming (NLP) is expert at building this on a communication level. That would be another whole book to explain though.

Once you see these techniques it is hard to unsee or unhear them. Take some time to research Edward Bernays's (Dr. Freud's nephew) propaganda work. It was used to revitalize the economy after the great depression in the 1930's. You will see how this style of influence changed America and then the world. It is extremely interesting reading to comprehend group think.

How does this information change how you view some of the social influence that has guided your decisions and buying options in the past. What will change for you in the future?

A FEW NATIONAL RESOURCES – CONNECT WITH US FOR REGIONAL OR LOCAL

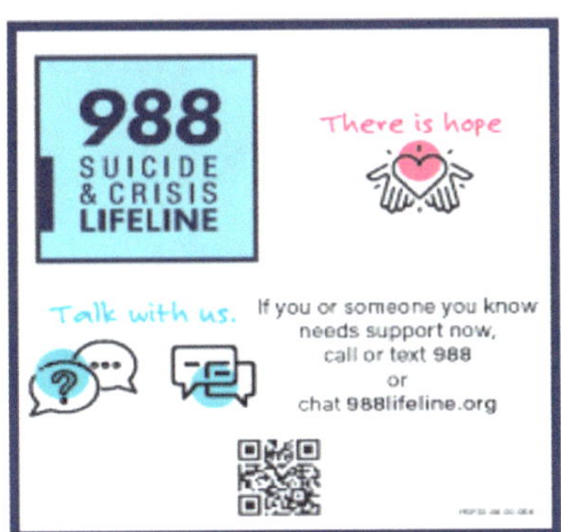

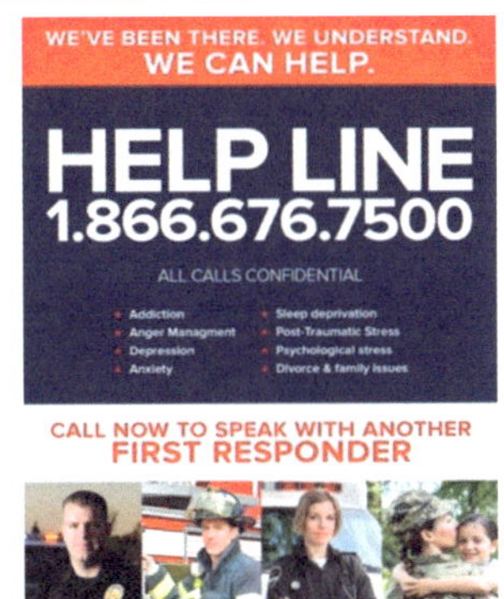

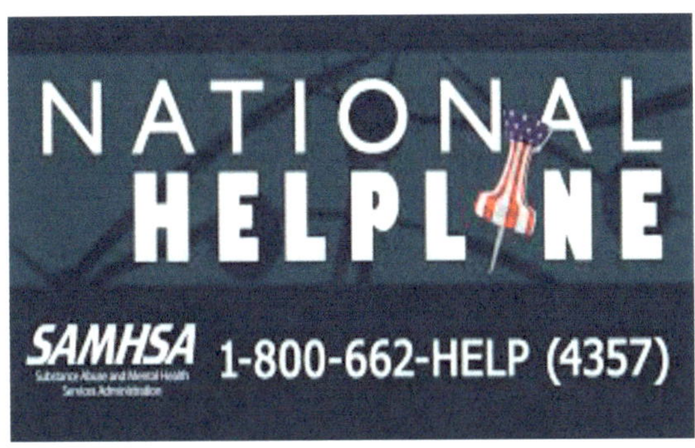

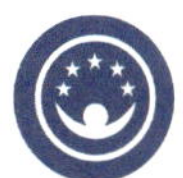

WRITTEN BY

American Addiction Centers

American Addiction Centers | national behavioral healthcare provider focused on addiction treatment. 800.466.8064

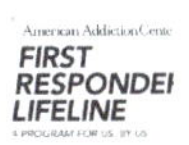

First Responders

Our counselors are always on-hand to assist you. Helpline Firefighters: 888–337–9381 Police Officers: 888–997–5675

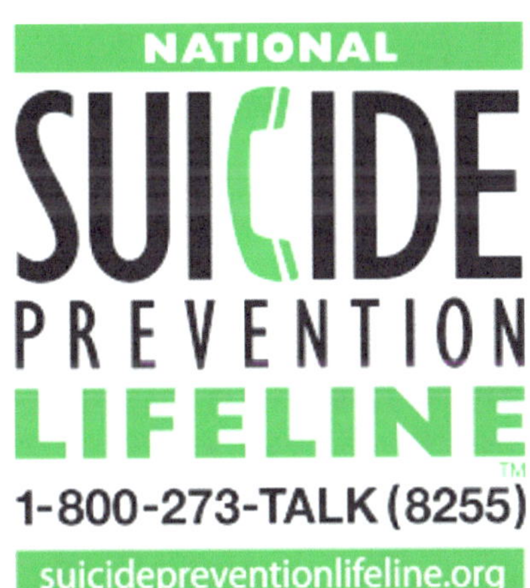

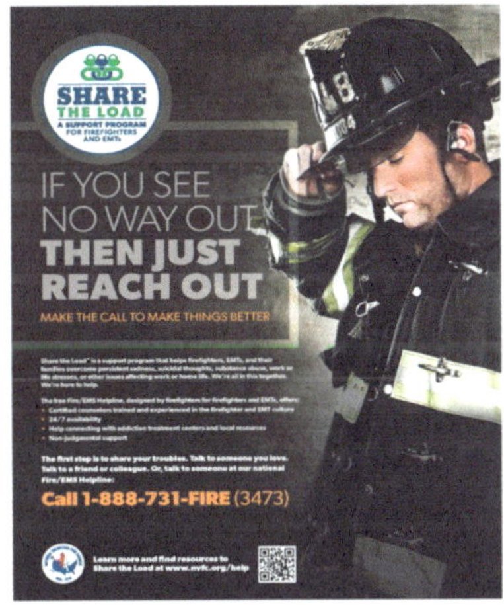

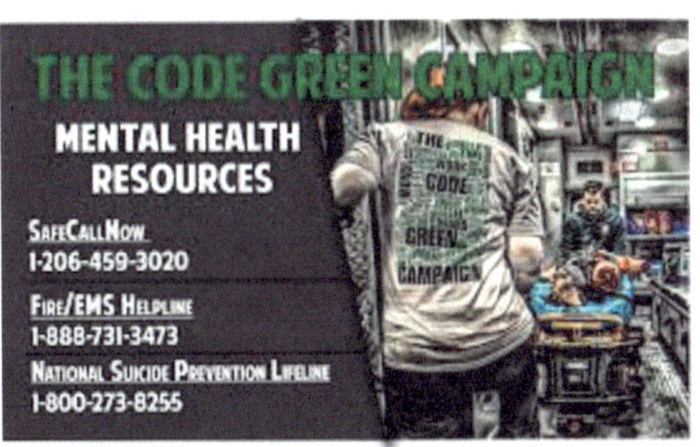

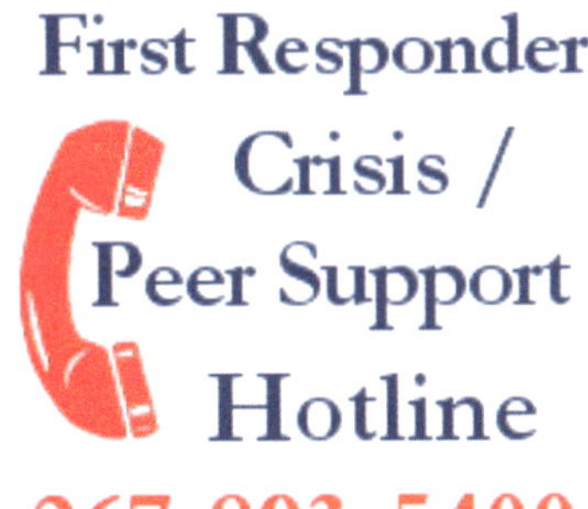

Your Customized Workshop *is a call away...*

1-844-444-GBTC (4282) | info@goingbeyondthecall.com

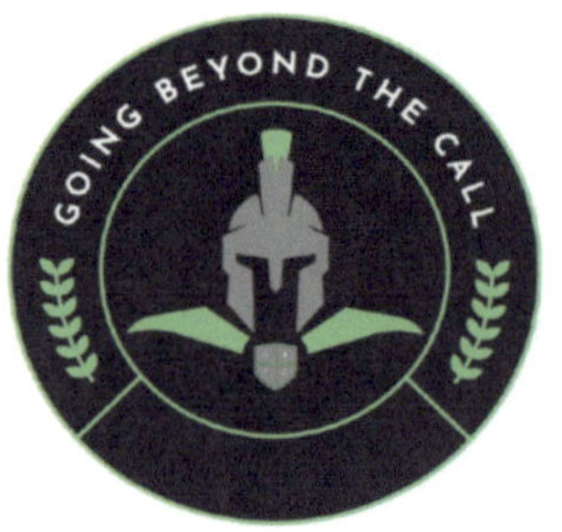

S.M.A.R.T.

SURVIVE THE MENTAL AMBUSH RESILIENCY TACTICS

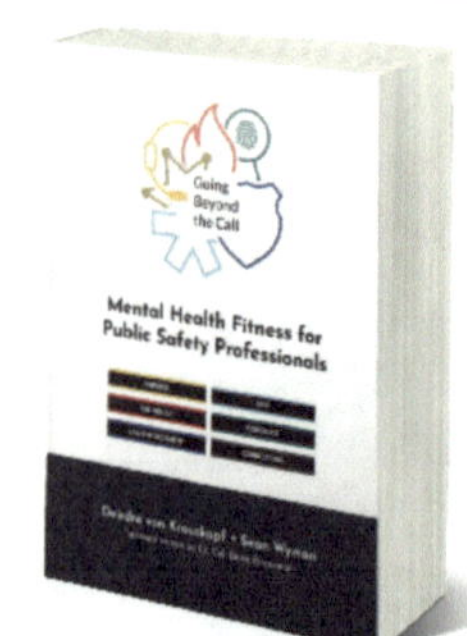

TRAUMA IMPACTS

Mental Ambush Preparedness

What you see, hear, and manage every shift has a guaranteed psychological, physiological, organizational, and relationship impact. From burnout, hyper-vigilance, to the more serious disorders and mental health challenges.

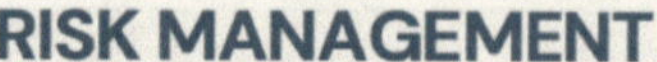

RISK MANAGEMENT

There is a significant organizational cost to stress injuries and maladaptive coping choices that are rarely measured, tracked or mitigated well. Our services will improve your bottom line.

ADAPTIVE RESILIENCY

These professions need to go beyond the bounce back factor.

Repeated vigilance, stress, psychological and moral injury require mental ambush preparedness. Our advanced recovery tools help avoid burnout, compassion fatigue, and the more damaging, and often unknown long term physical, and mental fitness impacts.

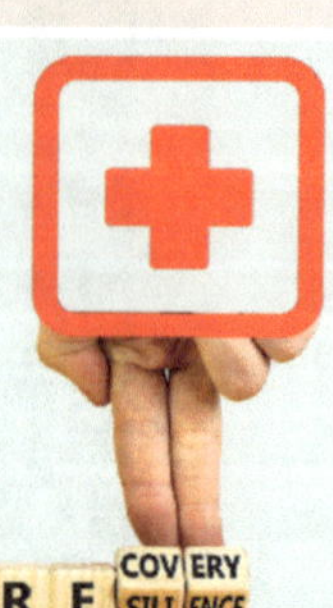

STRATEGIC COMMUNICATIONS

Your words, body language, biases, and approach matter. A pre-escalation mindset avoids emotionalized responses within you, and by those you are communicating with.

- Control Self
- Manage Interactions
- Influence Others to best outcome for all

VIGILANCE BALANCE

Grow adaptive situational awareness for managing interactions to gain the best outcome for all, and avoid being the next YouTube led persecution.

How to turn down the hyper-vigilance while remaining vigilant. How to use mindful resilience to transition from on-duty to off-duty to quickly reset the nervous system, improving health, sleep quality, and general life enjoyment.

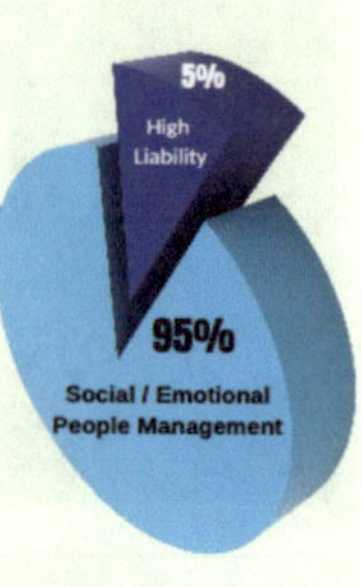

RELATIONSHIP MANAGEMENT

Protect those you love from the unimaginable things you manage without shutting down, pushing them away, or challenging trust.

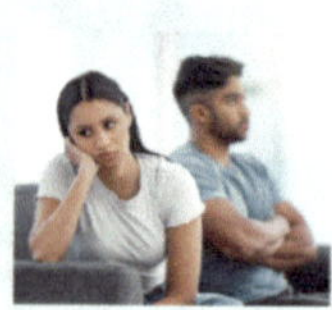

Develop peer communication strategies to ensure necessary team, family, and self-care protocols are in place.

EMOTIONAL INTELLIGENCE and EGO STATES

Learn why some more resilient and able to adapt to the daily stressors and challenges faced.

Beyond *mental health first aid;* we share how to develop oneself for added happiness, better brain and body wellness, improved relationships, and positive physical and mental health

On Going Beyond the Call
"You hold in your hands one of the most important books of our time.
A hidden impact, a stigmatized secret that overshadows the men and women who sacrifice every day."

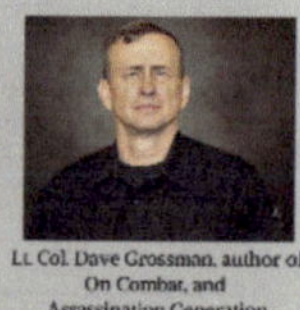

Lt. Col. Dave Grossman, author of On Combat, and Assassination Generation

Deirdre von Krauskopf | **Sean Wyman**
Going Beyond the Call LLC. **www.GBTC911.com. | gbtcbook.com**
844.411.4282 (411-GBTC) **info@GoingBeyondTheCall.com**

ABOUT THE AUTHORS

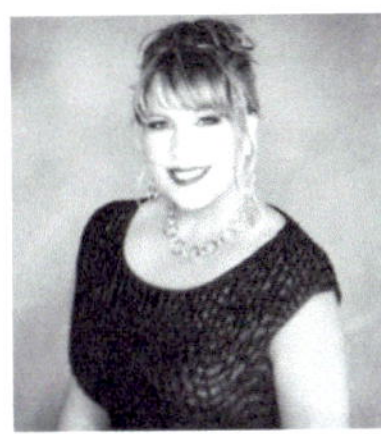

Deirdre von Krauskopf

Deirdre von Krauskopf developed a strong fortitude and resilience from necessity amid a traumatic childhood environment. A life in constant survival mode, abuse at home, severe bullying, and forced participation in gang life to fight for her safety between school and home. Almost every teacher, adult, and authority she faced prophesied she would be dead or in jail before reaching adulthood. Fighting became the one thing she excelled at, she took command at 14 and beaten savagely by her stepmother she resisted the violent urge to end another's life and ran away. Hiding in a friend's cement basement, she worked to pay her board and used the family church to find and negotiate a custody release to her mother a few months later by leveraging her silence, as speaking up would put her handicapped half-brother in the system, which isn't kind to challenged kids. Similar to many child victims, threats had kept her and her siblings quiet but there comes a time when you realize the only victor in silence is the abuser.

With the lessons of her past, she drove herself to success wanting to bury her past and forget. While parenting and funding her mother, she found a new family in Army Cadets at 14, full time Army Reserves at 17, and then marrying into the law enforcement family at 18 and working in that field. She attained her safe, secure, calm, loving home, locked her trauma in a vault and never looked back. With the addition of her son at 29 she was enjoying the best life could offer in career and family success until 26 years later when trauma came crashing in again, ripped open her locked vault and flooded her with challenges merged from past to present.

She had nursed her husband through so many injuries and sleepless nights, together, they had always been okay. He had many near miss accidents, threats to him and our family by hardened criminals, even shot at but then one time, the last near-death incident hit harder. Slowly the man she loved stopped coming home and the stranger in his place set off her long-vaulted childhood triggers. It was devastating to be a top of her field human behavior "fixer" who failed her most important role. The unquiet in her head returned, unable to find a way to close the growing divide and no longer feeling safe, secure, or calm, her crushed soul ran away once more. Needing to understand she educated herself in psychology and PTSD, found training to develop herself further and combined education and life experience vowing to make a difference for other public safety professional families.

Her career spans Military, Law Enforcement, Senior Operational and Strategic Project Management. With a passionate drive to serve others Deirdre has developed her expertise in Human Behavior, Neuroscience, Emotional Intelligence, Body Language, Trauma-Informed Care and Strategic Communications. She helps individuals and organizations achieve measurable, transformational change utilizing brain and behavioral sciences. She has written 5 books and over 50 training programs.

CHECK OUT DEIRDRE'S LEADERSHIP BOOK: MISTAKENLY UNDERAPPRECIATED ~ A GUIDE FOR TURING AROUND TOXIC AND CHALLENGING WORK ENVIORNMENTS

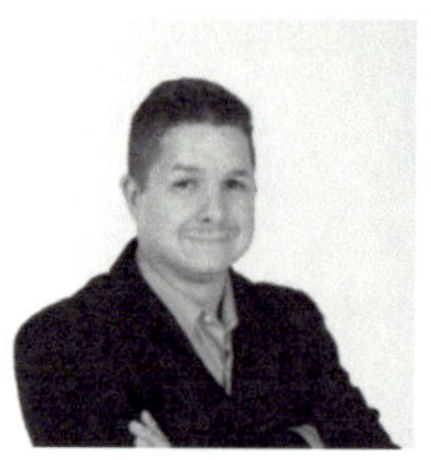

Sean Wyman

Sean grew up in poverty within the suburbs of Washington DC as a young child of an interracial relationship heated with underlying racial tension. Bullied as a minority, he is highly empathetic to generational and racial trauma of all kinds. Fighting for survival from a violent addicted and abusive drug dealing stepfather Sean was quickly forced to learn how to manage daily mental and physical abuse. He adapted to survive using the streets as his guide. After three years of continual abuse, he came close to a fatal decision, to take his stepfathers life, instead he left the gun at the end of the bed running away and changing his life forever.

His mother said he couldn't come back, and he was forced into a life of foster care and group homes, facing new problems along with old ones that were never resolved. Sean went from being bullied to becoming the bully. By the time he was a teenager, he had discovered damaging coping mechanisms to numb his pain. Ones that he became addicted to, and controlled by, for several years. A military Veteran with the Army Rangers, a Law Enforcement Officer with experience in many specialty units he kept swallowing down and pushing away the darkness. For over thirty years Sean's secret past was hidden in a vault while he privately suffered from denial, regret, anger, misery, and anxiety. It destroyed his first marriage and left him drowning in debt. The catalyst which pushed him to be a better man for his beautiful wife and family today. This influx of goodness was the turning point in his life that at first, he thought was just for him, but soon realized it was meant for millions of others like him.

Now, as the best-selling author and a noted speaker he promotes his passion for serving others. Sean achieved a certification in Trauma-Informed Care and further as a Trauma-Informed Professional. Sean is also a licensed provider of Verbal Aikido, a program of strategic communications, emotional intelligence, and the philosophy of Aikido, staying calm, controlled, and balanced in the moment. Sean has been street testing these tactics for years and making a significant impact in the community he serves with positive feedback from his partners and peers. Sean reached out to Deirdre to combine their work, together they created a program to save the many public safety folks battling the same mental ambush and enhance all lives in the process. After Sean 'street tested' the work they wrote Going Beyond the Call.

Today an 18+ year Law Enforcement Officer and Trainer, Army Ranger Veteran, father of 3, and husband of 14 years, Sean shares his story, the lessons learned, and most importantly teaches others as a trauma-informed care speaker, facilitator, and bestselling author with one purpose; help others realize that to them what is impossible with the right M.O.V.E.M.E.N.T. is possible. Sean is passionate about serving his brothers and sisters with the ground-breaking book, Going Beyond the Call because he has seen and battle-tested the contents and knows the benefits first-hand. His mission is to turn the increasingly devastating trend of suicides, PTSD, and relationship failures within the ranks of the public safety professions. Everyone is calling for an answer ... THIS is the solution!

CHECK OUT SEAN'S BEST-SELLING BOOK: LET GO: THE MOVEMENT PROCESS

INDEX

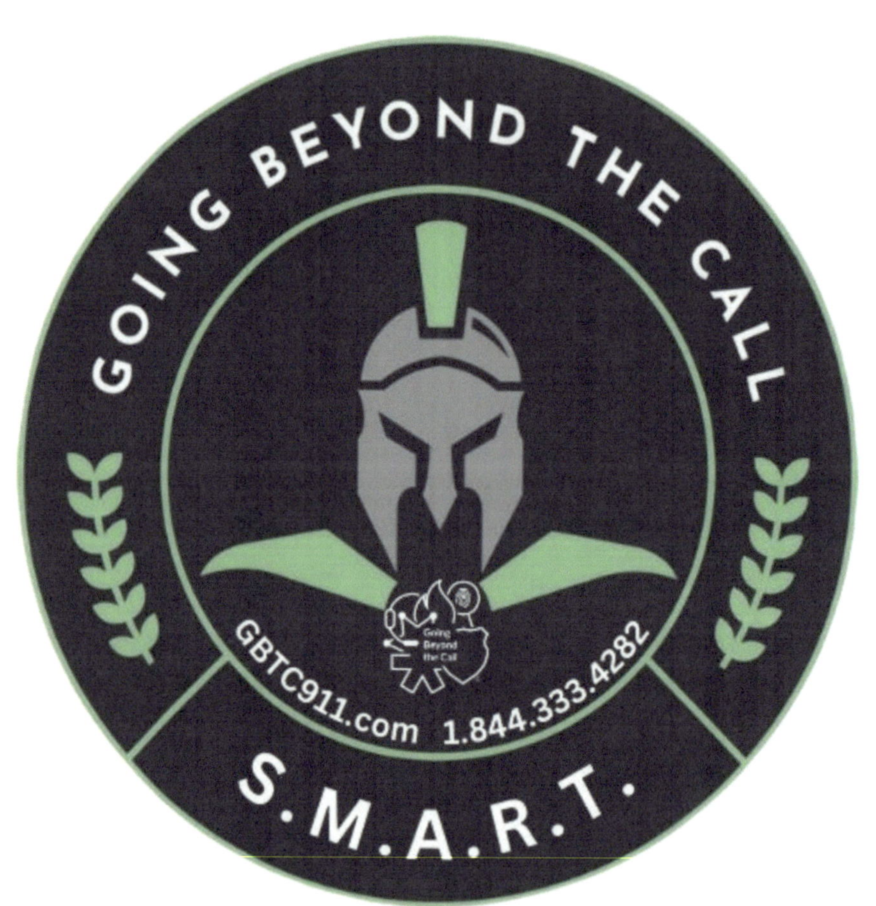
GOING BEYOND THE CALL
GBTC911.com 1.844.333.4282
S.M.A.R.T.

Made in the USA
Columbia, SC
06 November 2023